The Dynamics of Atherosclerosis

John B Duguid CBE MD

The Dynamics of Atherosclerosis

Professor Emeritus of Pathology in the University of Newcastle-upon-Tyne. Formerly Professor of Pathology and Bacteriology in the Welsh National School of Medicine, Cardiff

Aberdeen University Press

First published 1976
© John B Duguid 1976
ISBN   0 900015 36 5
Printed in Great Britain
by the Aberdeen University Press

Contents

Foreword

By A. S. Douglas
Regius Professor of Medicine, University of Aberdeen

It is a unique privilege to write the foreword to this monograph by Professor J B Duguid.

In North America and to a lesser extent in Western Europe enormous financial and human resources have been expended in the pursuit of fundamental knowledge on arterial disease: some have studied the arterial wall, others the constituents of the occluding thrombus. During the last two decades the appropriate literature has been flooded by contributions in this area of clinical and scientific endeavour. Studies have been carried out on the vessel wall, platelets, the coagulation mechanism and the fibrinolytic enzyme system.

These endeavours have ranged from well designed clinical trials to sophisticated biochemistry and electron microscopy. The area of interest for the individual investigator has become narrower, as more information has accumulated. A team of biochemists is required to make a small new advance in the molecular structure of fibrinogen; whole biological departments are needed to make additions to the established data on the properties of the platelet membrane. To run the trial of a drug evaluating secondary prevention in survivors of myocardial infarction needs the collaboration of twenty hospital centres and the expenditure of one million pounds or two million dollars.

The author, a youthful octogenarian, lives in retirement, surrounded by friends in Bieldside, Aberdeen. There are few, with such unrivalled academic reputation, who can stand back from the problem of arterial disease and take a broad view. Such a man is Jack Duguid. He has the vision to restate and enlarge upon a long forgotten viewpoint.

Many will lift this monograph and fail to read it because they will conclude that this is a repetition of the thrombogenic theory of atheroma; Professor Duguid has of course made important scientific contributions on that theme; in this book however, it receives only brief mention. In the field of medical scientific endeavour there is an adage that there are few original discoveries, merely repetitions of earlier findings; when theories or facts are restated the observer often only then re-explores the literature establishing that an experimental finding or an hypothesis has been recorded previously. Professor Duguid's reputation in the field is often linked to his reappraisal of the Rokitansky thrombogenic theory of atheroma, first postulated in the middle of the nineteenth century. On this occasion the author has used as a starting point the observations of one of his teachers Professor J A MacWilliam, formerly Professor of Physiology in this University. Professor Duguid has set down important new concepts on the aetiology of the common illness of our times.

Introduction

In the early 1920s, while embarking on a study of atheroma of the aorta, I came across a communication by J. A. MacWilliam (1902) on the elasticity of arteries in which he pointed out that in excised vessels elasticity is influenced by post-mortem contraction, as are also, incidentally, the histological appearances. Impelled by my admiration for MacWilliam as a teacher in my own medical school and an outstanding investigator, I read the communication with special interest, and it is well that I did so as it gave me an insight into an aspect of arterial pathology which most writers on the subject seem to have overlooked.

MacWilliam showed that the arteries remain alive and contract after the death of the individual, the contraction often being maintained for several days, with the result that most of the arteries we study in histological sections are more or less contracted, and this affects their appearance. He also noted that the degree of post-mortem contraction is variable, depending on such factors as the age of the individual, the tone of the arteries at death and the length of time that has elapsed since death. These factors produce wide variations in histological appearances, and it seemed to me that this must be of importance in the interpretation of arterial lesions, yet it was notable that no writer on the subject at that time either mentioned post-mortem contractions or referred to MacWilliam's work.

In the early 1920s the pathology of atheroma had undergone a radical change. Most early writers had viewed the lesions as a form of mechanical disruption caused by excessive pulse movements, but in 1913 the Russian workers Anitschkow and Chalatow showed that lipid deposits resembling atheroma could be produced in the rabbit aorta by the oral administration of cholesterol and from then on the attention of pathologists was turned almost with one accord to the study of lipids. Atheroma then came to be regarded as a fatty infiltration of the arteries due to a disordered lipid metabolism, and mechanical considerations were discarded and to a large extent forgotten.

During the last thirty years a vast literature has accumulated on the subject of atheroma, or atherosclerosis as it is now called, and is concerned almost exclusively with lipids and the dangers of fatty foods. The function and behaviour of arteries are seldom referred to and, incredible though it may seem, pulse movements are hardly ever mentioned in relation to arterial pathology. This is remarkable in view of the fact that the aorta and its main branches, where pulse movements are most extensive, are the vessels most subject to atherosclerosis, and it is hard to believe that these movements can be totally dissociated from the lesions.

This state of affairs cannot be regarded as satisfactory and the time has surely come for a fresh assessment of the problem. We can no longer look on arteries as if they were rigid tubes, which is virtually what we are doing when we ignore pulse movements. My purpose in this monograph is to re-introduce the older mechanical theory along with some fresh information showing how, when the lesions are studied with movements in mind, many of the features which have in the past seemed inexplicable can be understood. It then becomes clear that, underlying the fatty changes and mostly concealed by them, there is a far more destructive lesion of a kind which almost certainly denotes a mechanical disruption such as the early observers recognised. This is not to say that pulsation is directly the cause of atherosclerosis. The more likely cause, as I suggested many years ago, is stiffening of the intima by fibrous or other thickenings interfering with the pulse movements and leading to discord and disruption in the vessel wall.

In the following chapters I shall endeavour to bring together evidence which has convinced me that atherosclerotic lesions are foci of disruption and haemorrhage due to loss of flexibility of the intima, and that fatty deposits call for no metabolic explanation but are simply products of shed blood, as Winternitz and his co-workers long ago suggested. This, it will be understood, is a matter of no small importance since on it must depend our approach to the problem of prevention. Must we continue to treat atherosclerosis as a metabolic disorder, or should we revert to the views of the early observers and regard it as a mechanical lesion due to a disturbance of arterial function?

My interest all along has been mainly in the study of mural thrombi and the part they play in the pathogenesis of atherosclerosis but in the last twenty years my attention has been drawn especially to the microthrombi, those minute surface encrustations which form on artery walls and which are only now beginning to receive the recognition they deserve. It is to my lasting regret that time and circumstances did not allow me to follow that line of investigation further as I believe it is there that the secret of the ageing process is to be found.

To have a clear understanding of the mechanical concept it is necessary to recognise certain peculiarities in the structure and functions of the arterial walls not usually given much prominence in the textbooks but clearly brought out in MacWilliam's work. Accordingly a first chapter will be devoted to an analysis of the elastic properties of arteries, an understanding of which is of prime importance in the interpretation of arterial lesions.

To students much of the difficulty in arterial pathology is in the terminology. Such terms as atheroma, atherosclerosis and arteriosclerosis and their application to the different parts of the arterial system can be confusing, whilst the change from atheroma to atherosclerosis, like so many other reforms in medical terminology, has added nothing to our understanding of the condition. I share Sir George Pickering's dislike of the new term with its emphasis on the fatty component of the lesion, but I have nevertheless felt compelled to use it since it is the one commonly understood the world over, and to use any other would be to risk further confusion. For convenience I use the term atheroma in reference to earlier works and atherosclerosis to the more modern, taking the two as synonymous, although that was obviously not in Marchand's mind when he introduced the newer term.

Chapter One

Functional Considerations

Arterial pathology has been bedevilled in the past by a strange lack of agreement on the simple question whether or not the arteries move in pulsation. Lister once wrote: 'If a surgeon exposes an artery he does not find that he is dealing with a body that swells with every pulse, but with one of unvaring dimensions', and this has been quoted as justification for leaving pulse movements out of account in interpreting arterial lesions. That some writers should have taken this way of avoiding an awkward problem is understandable, but that almost every one of the vast numbers who have written on arterial diseases in the last half century should have seen fit to ignore pulse movements altogether seems tantamount to denying their existence and calls for a reassessment of the situation.

Pulse Movements

In the healthy young adult 60 ml or more of blood are thrust into the aorta with every heart beat and that vessel, not being a rigid tube, yields and enlarges to accommodate the additional volume but, being elastic, contracts again to its former size when the blood is passed on. Thus, no matter whether the aorta enlarges by lengthening or by dilatation, its walls and also those of its main branches must stretch and contract with each heart beat, and in the following chapters it will be shown how these movements can be the determining factors in the development of atherosclerosis. To understand this, however, it is necessary first to consider in some detail the special structure of the arterial walls. These are elastic, but they must not be thought of as homogeneous structures since they are composed of several tissues, muscle, elastic tissue, collagen, etc., which differ widely in their elasticity, and to understand atherosclerosis one must know something of how these tissues behave in relation to one another in pulsation. It is necessary, therefore, before approaching the pathology of the artery walls, to devote this section to a consideration of their functional properties.

Much information on the arterial pulse can be found in the writings of Wiggers (1928), McDonald (1964) and others but it is difficult to obtain exact information on the degrees of stretching the various arteries undergo in pulsation. What we do know is that the force responsible for the stretching is generated in the heart and is therefore greatest in the proximal part of the arterial system and diminishes in strength as the distance from the heart increases. Consequently pulse movements are likely to be greatest in the aorta and its main branches and less, or absent, in the peripheral arteries. This, no doubt, explains why some of the peripheral arteries do not, as Lister pointed out, seem to 'swell at every pulse beat' and, incidentally, why the peripheral arteries do not as a rule become atherosclerotic. It is in the aorta and its main branches, where pulse movements are at their maximum, that atherosclerosis mainly develops. The movements may be slight but, considering that they recur something like a hundred thousand times a day without respite throughout life, it is easy to appreciate how they can be a source of what the early writers called 'wear and tear'.

Elasticity in Arteries

Since arteries contain muscle the question of a muscular contraction with each pulse beat has been considered, but generally rejected. It is assumed that the function of the medial muscle is to control the mean diameter of the artery, whilst pulse movements are determined by alterations in pressure produced by the ventricular contractions. At systole the pressure in the proximal arteries is raised and these vessels, being elastic, yield and enlarge but recoil again to their former size when the pressure falls. Thus, it is their elasticity* that enables them to maintain an even mean calibre and, as we shall see, it is loss of elasticity that accounts for most of the pathological changes we have to consider.

Attempts have been made to measure the elasticity of arteries by

* Elasticity in arteries is a somewhat confused subject because, as Burton (1967) points out, the meaning of the term is doubtful. Elasticity, as commonly understood refers to that quality which enables a material to be stretched while retaining its ability to spring back to its former shape when the stretching force is removed, but this is not the technical meaning. Elasticity in physics, as Burton explains, is the property by which a material resists deformation, developing an opposing elastic tension. In this sense steel has a higher coefficient of elasticity than rubber, and a sclerotic artery a higher elasticity than a normal one: which is not as we understand it. In arteries the properties we have to consider are stretchability, or distensibility and resilience, and these are generally understood under the term elasticity, which is the one we shall mostly use.

suspending weights to strips of excised vessel walls and plotting their extensibility curves or by inflating lengths of excised vessels and recording their distensibility under rising pressures, but the fallacy of such records was brought to light by MacWilliam. He showed that the elasticity of excised arteries depends, not on the so-called 'elastic tissue' in their walls but on the degree of post-mortem contraction in their muscle, which is variable, contracted arteries having a greater degree of stretchability and resilience than relaxed ones.

Post-mortem Contraction

In the proceedings of the Royal Society of 1902 and in a more accessible communication published in collaboration with Mackie in 1908, MacWilliam showed that arteries retain their vitality for three or four days after the death of the individual and will continue to contract in response to various stimuli such as cooling, exposure

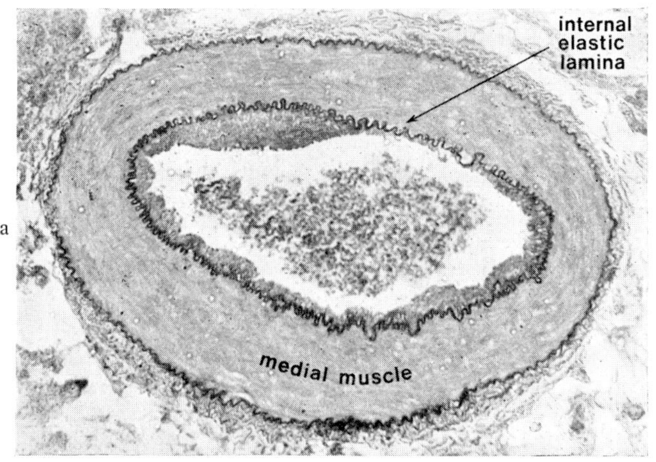

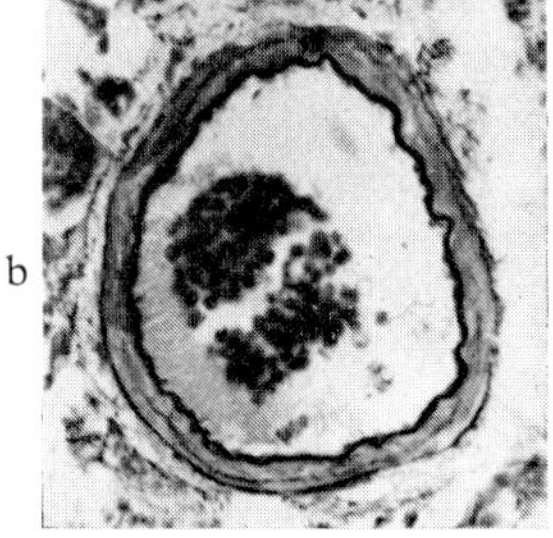

FIG. 1. Effects of post-mortem contraction: paraffin sections, Weigert's elastic tissue stain. (a) A strongly contracted artery, thick walled with deeply wrinkled elastic lamina. (b) A smaller artery in which post-mortem contraction has passed off, widely dilated, and then walled with elastic lamina more nearly straightened.

to air, alcohol, formol etc. and remain contracted for some days. This means that the arteries we study in sections are in a more or less contracted state, which notably affects their appearance, contracted arteries being thick walled and narrow, with deeply wavy elastic laminae (fig 1a) whilst relaxed ones are thin walled and wide, with their elastic laminae more nearly straightened (fig 1b).

MacWilliam and Mackie explained that the degree of post-mortem contraction varies, depending on the tone of the muscle at death, being strongly marked in the healthy young animal which has been killed suddenly and weak in the individual who has died after a long illness. They showed that the contraction can be abolished by exposure to certain chemicals such as sodium fluoride or ammonia vapour, and that without such interference it naturally passes off in time. Consequently, in tissues which have been long dead before fixation the arteries may appear thin walled and widely dilated. MacWilliam and Mackie were mainly concerned with the elasticity of the arteries but, to the histo-pathologist, their more important contribution was the demonstration of how post-mortem contraction affects histological appearances. Failure to appreciate this has undoubtedly resulted in misconceptions: for example, arteries which appear thick walled in section have sometimes been taken to be hypertrophic, whereas they merely showed strong post-mortem contraction. Similarly the ratio of wall thickness to lumen diameter has been used retrospectively as an index of circulatory effectiveness, whereas it simply depends on the degree of post-mortem contraction. But most important of all has been the almost universal failure to appreciate how post-mortem contraction affects histological appearances in arteries.

Elastic Tissue

Some confusion regarding the elasticity of arteries arises from the fact that one of the components of the arterial wall is called elastic tissue. Since this is more plentiful in the aorta than in other vessels, the aorta is called an 'elastic artery' which has led to the belief that it is functionally more stretchable and resilient than other arteries. MacWilliam and Mackie found that the aorta was less stretchable and resilient than the peripheral arteries, and that the arteries with most muscle in their walls were the most elastic. Moreover, they found that the distensibility of an artery increases with the degree of post-mortem contraction, which was to be expected since contracted muscle has further to stretch before reaching the limit of its extensibility than has relaxed, or stretched muscle.

Some years ago, in collaboration with Dr Jo Boissard, the writer tested the distensibility and resilience of various excised arteries, human and animal, by inflating them with improvised balloons. Although the measurements obtained were too erratic to be worth reporting, it was learned that the aorta had a low initial resistance to distension but a very short range of distensibility, whereas the peripheral, or so-called 'muscular arteries' had a relatively high initial resistance to distension but could nevertheless be inflated to two or three times their initial diameters and still return, albeit slowly, to their former size when the pressure was released. From these findings it was inferred that it is to the muscle rather than to the elastic tissue that the arteries owe their resilience, and that muscle is in fact the more elastic of the two tissues. Cook, Salmo and Yates (1975) have noted that the internal elastic lamina does not increase in length when an artery is distended but merely changes its shape. Shennan used to teach that the so-called elastic laminae were relatively tough structures acting as check cords preventing overdistension of the arteries.

Arrangement of Tissues

There is, however, no need to inflate arteries to get an indication of the relative elasticity of the various components of their walls, as this is clearly enough shown by the arrangement of the elastic laminae in most histological sections. The fact that they are wavy in section shows that in post-mortem contraction they are unable to shorten to the same extent as the vessel wall as a whole and so have to become wrinkled in order to comply with the contraction.*

* It has been suggested that the wavy form of the elastic laminae represents a special quality like that of a coiled spring but, while something like this is perhaps imaginable in the aorta, where the arrangement of the elastic laminae in the media has been likened to that of a spring mattress, it would be hard to imagine that the wrinkling of the internal elastic lamina in the artery shown in fig 1a, for example, provided the force responsible for the contraction of that vessel. Clearly it is the resilience of the medial muscle that is responsible for the recoil of the vessel wall when the stretching force is reduced.

The reader by now may well be questioning what all this has to do with atherosclerosis, and the answer is that it provides a clue to the problem. From studies of the elastic laminae two principles emerge: first, that not all the components of the vessel wall are equally elastic, and secondly, that those of lesser elasticity conform to contractions beyond their elastic range by bending or wrinkling. This is most clearly shown by the elastic laminae, and hence our interest in them, but they are not the only components to which the principle applies. In the aorta and its main branches there is in the intima a variable amount of fibrous (collagenous) tissue which is probably even less resilient than the elastic tissue. In young arteries it consists of thin fibres which are loosely arranged and flexible so that they can easily comply with movements but, with increasing age and in pathological conditions, a fibrous tissue of a denser and less flexible type makes its appearance in the intima and, as we shall see, it is the failure of this tissue to comply normally with pulse movements that accounts for the disruption, haemorrhage and fatty changes that constitute atheroma.

Chapter Two

Atherosclerosis

This lesion, which used to be called atheroma, is characterised by nodular fibrous thickenings of the intima with fatty change. It occurs mostly in the aorta and its main branches, especially the coronary arteries, the basal arteries of the brain and sometimes in the pulmonary arteries in cases of pulmonary hypertension. It is one of the commonest of human lesions and has been described countless times, so that a further systematic account of it here would be superfluous. There are, however, certain features which are commonly overlooked and to which attention needs to be called.

Effects of Post-mortem Contraction

It is sometimes noted that when a severely atheromatous aorta is slit open lengthwise in the usual way and laid flat, it tends to curl backwards so that the intima is on the convex surface (fig 2). How this is brought about is seen when the artery is viewed in section. In post-mortem contraction the thickened part of the intima, being too stiff to contract to the same extent as the subjacent media,

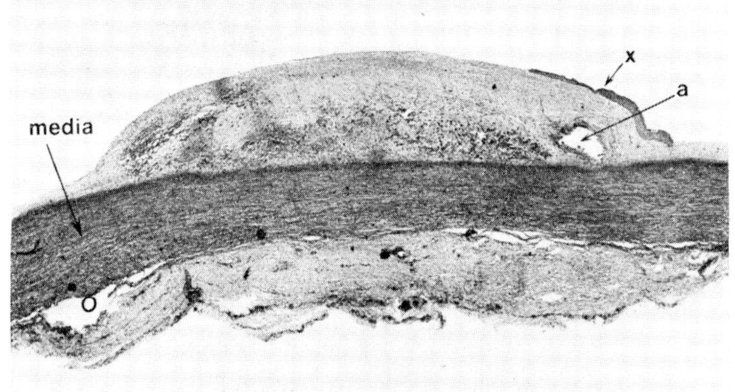

FIG. 2. Aortic atherosclerosis as commonly represented, the aorta having been slit open and laid flat. A fibrous thickening of the intima has reduced the flexibility of that coat so that it is less shortened than the media and the curvature of the wall is reversed. The thickening has also reduced to some extent the contraction of the subjacent part of the media so that there is thinning at that part. Very little fat is present except a small focus of atheroma at a, the lesion being an example of Montgomery's 'hard atheroma' or what is sometimes called a pearly plaque. The dark layer at x is a micro-thrombus. Frozen section: Sudan III and haemalum, ×8.

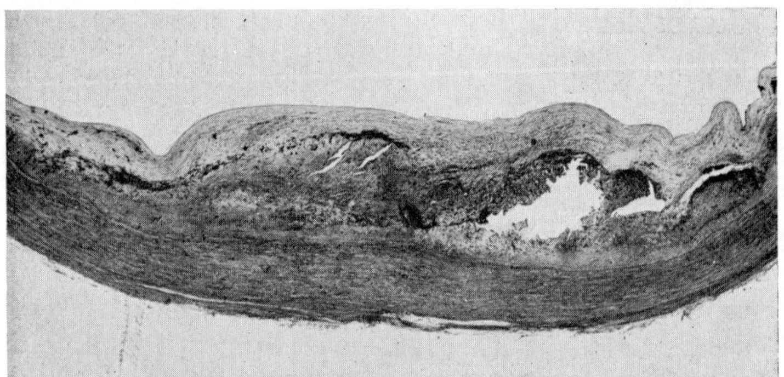

FIG. 3. Aortic atherosclerosis shown in its natural shape. Post-mortem contraction has crumpled the stiffened intima so that the inner layers are partly split away from the outer ones and the spaces between filled with fatty debris, an example of Montgomery's 'soft atheroma'. Frozen section: Sudan III and haemalum, ×8.

remains more or less expanded, so that it forms a wider arc and the curve of the wall at that part is consequently reversed. If, on the other hand, the vessel wall is fixed and hardened in formalin before being opened, its natural cylindrical shape is preserved and the thickened intima is then forced to conform to post-mortem contraction by crumpling or buckling (fig 3), so that its deeper layers are loosened and torn apart. Spaces are thus formed in the intima and these, becoming filled with fatty debris, constitute atheroma.

The Mechanical Theory

These observations prompted the writer in 1926 to suggest that atheroma was a mechanical effect due to stiffening of the intima. It seemed that if the artery walls stretch and recoil in pulsation, no matter whether the movements involve dilatation and contraction or lengthening and shortening of the vessels, failure of any part of the intima to comply with these movements must result in discord and disruption of the kind seen in atheroma. This was but a modification of the old mechanical theory which originated with Virchow and which was still current in the early part of this century. Allbutt (1915) in England and Aschoff (1924) in Germany considered that atheromatous lesions were mechanical tears due to shearing effects with the sliding of one layer of the intima over another in excessive pulse movements. The new suggestion was that the tears were due not to excessive movements but to failure of the stiffened intima to comply with the normal movements of pulsation.

Diagram I

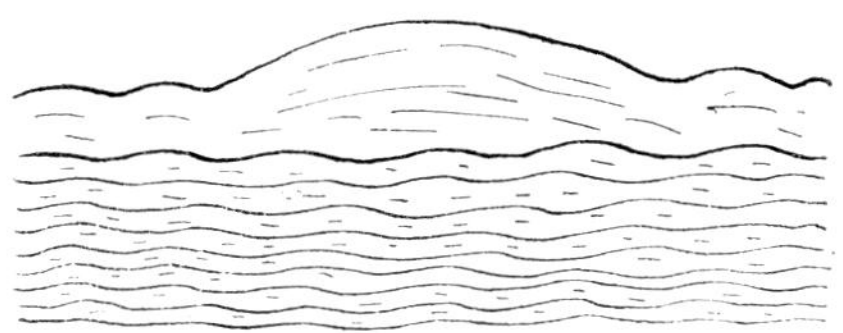

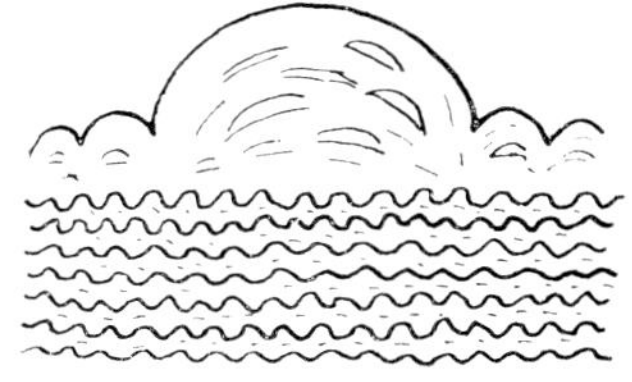

Diagram II

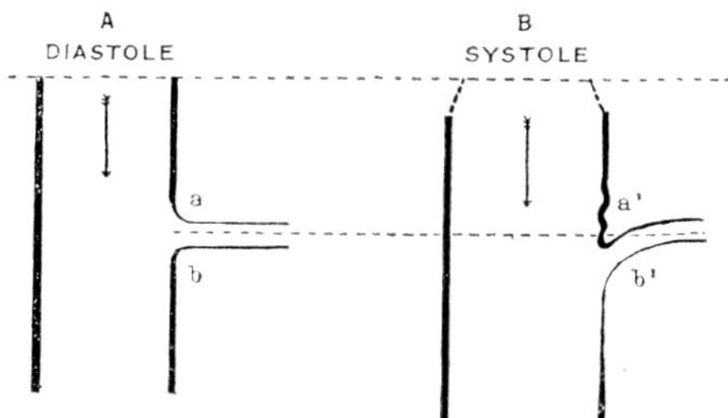

In the communication of 1926 the two diagrams, here reproduced, were included to illustrate the effects of movements, diagram 1 showing the effect of local thickening of the intima. Diagram 2 explains the predilection of atheroma for areas around branches and bifurcations. Where, for example, the intercostal arteries leave the aorta they are partly anchored to bony structures and, if we assume that the aorta lengthens and shortens in pulsation, it will follow that in certain phases of the pulse cycle certain parts of the vessel wall will be stretched abnormally far to compensate for reduced stretching in other parts.

Nothing, so far as the writer has seen, has come to light that invalidates the suggestion put forward in 1926, nevertheless the suggestion excited little interest since it was based on a post-mortem appearance the interpretation of which was open to question. It was doubtful if in life an artery could ever contract to the same extent as it could after death when no longer distended with blood, and it was questionable if pulse movements could ever be strong enough or extensive enough to tear the tissues in the way suggested. Moreover the suggestion contributed little of value since it did not explain how either of the two main features of atherosclerosis, namely the fibrous thickenings of the intima or the fatty changes are produced. We now have answers to these questions and they are revealed on pages 13 and 48, but they are best understood if we follow the investigation step by step so as to bring out the line of reasoning on which they are based.

The Overgrowth Theory

Ever since the advent of Virchow's 'cellular theory' it has been taken for granted that the fibrous thickenings in atheroma are overgrowths, or proliferations of the intimal connective tissue cells excited by the presence of the fats. They look like overgrowths and there seems no reason to think otherwise but for one consideration – in the coronary arteries they are sometimes associated with narrowing and occlusion, and it is difficult to see how in the wall of a pulsating artery a growth of fibrous tissue can lead to narrowing.

Arteries are elastic tubes supporting a high internal pressure of blood which tends always to distend them. At every rise in pulse pressure they yield and dilate but, being elastic, recoil again to their former size when the pressure subsides, so that they maintain an even mean diameter. The dilatation, it will be understood, is a passive movement imposed on them by the pulse pressure, but the recoil depends entirely on their own resilience and anything which impairs this property must leave them to some extent permanently dilated. Fibrous thickenings of the intima undoubtedly reduce their resilience and in most cases actually do lead to dilatation, but there are those important exceptions, occurring especially in the coronary arteries, where intimal thickenings encroach on the lumina and narrow them to the point of occlusion. The question how narrowing of the arteries is brought about has long troubled pathologists and was no doubt in Thoma's mind when he sought by his classical experiment to show that in life intimal thickenings did not encroach on the lumina of the arteries but bulged outwards.

Thoma's Experiment

Thoma noted that in the atheromatous aorta the medial coat subjacent to thickened plaques was often thinner than elsewhere (figs 2, 23 and 26) and he inferred therefrom that the muscle was weakened at those parts. He suggested that atheroma was the mark of a focal degeneration of the medial muscle with a giving way and outwards bulging of the vessel wall, followed by a compensatory proliferation of the intima filling in the bulge, and certainly the appearances in fig 26 seem to lend support to this idea. Thoma regarded the apparent encroachment of intimal thickenings into the lumina of arteries as an illusion caused by post-mortem contraction and, to prove this, he distended atheromatous aortas in cadavers with molten paraffin wax under pressure and, allowing the wax to harden, showed that the plaque bulged outwards instead of inwards, leaving the intimal surface smooth and even.

This seemed to support his contention that atheroma was due to a weakening of the media, but Thoma seems to have overlooked the fact that stretching of an artery wall involves thinning of the media. In atherosclerosis the fibrous thickenings of the intima tend to interfere with post-mortem contraction, clamping the affected parts of the artery in the more or less expanded position so that the medial coat subjacent to the larger fibrous plaques (fig 2), is commonly stretched thinner than at other parts. Thus, thinning of the media is an effect rather than a cause of atheroma.

Chapter Three

The Thrombogenic Hypothesis

The answer to the first of the two questions posed on page 10, relating to how fibrous thickenings of the intima are produced, is embodied in what has been called the thrombogenic hypothesis. It is easy in the light of that hypothesis to see that intimal thickenings with narrowing of arteries can be produced by thrombosis. A thrombus occupying the lumen of an artery is likely to reduce it and, when a mural thrombus becomes organised, it looks like a fibrous overgrowth of the intima. But in the 1920s thrombosis in the larger arteries was regarded as rare. It was supposed that the blood flow in these vessels was too rapid for thrombi to form, and evidence of a more than usually compelling character would have been required to persuade pathologists that intimal thickenings in the aorta could be organised thrombi, or that thrombosis played a part in so common a condition as atheroma. It was by a fortunate mischance that such evidence eventually came to light.

The Evidence

For several years sections of a thrombosed coronary artery were used in our pathology classes in the Welsh National School of Medicine to illustrate the principles of organisation. This vessel, which had a canalised thrombus in its lumen similar to that shown in fig 4, had provided sections for many years until the supply suddenly gave out. In a practical class which the writer was conducting some of the students indicated that they were unable to see what was being described and, on going to their assistance, it was found that in their sections the picture had changed. The technician in cutting the sections had unwittingly gone beyond the occluded part and, instead of an organised thrombus, the sections showed a patent artery with a greatly thickened intima in which there were all the characters of atherosclerosis, similar to that shown in fig 5.

On recalling the set of sections and arranging them in serial order it could be seen that the fibrous tissue which formed the thickened intima as shown in fig 5, was continuous with that which formed the canalised thrombus as seen in fig 4. In other words, the thrombus was not confined to the occluded part but extended

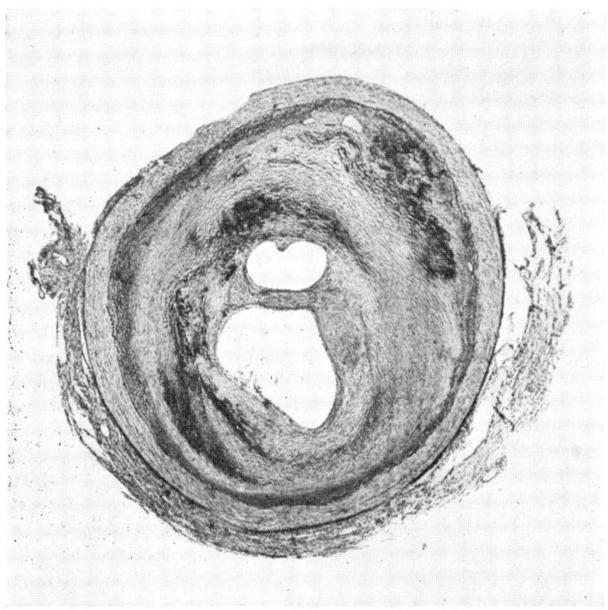

FIG. 4. Canalised thrombus in coronary artery. The lumen is occupied by an organised thrombus in which there are two endothelial-lined channels. The fibrous tissue between them is practically indistinguishable from that of the surrounding intima. The darker streaks in both the thrombus and the intima are fatty deposits. Frozen section: Sudan III and haemalum, × 20.

further along the artery as a thick inner lining which, being covered with endothelium, was incorporated into the intima and, being fibrous and fatty, had the characters of atherosclerosis. Thus came to light the little-known principle that, *when a mural thrombus forms in an artery it becomes covered with endothelium so that it is incorporated into the vessel wall and, when organised, forms a fibrous thickening of the intima* (Duguid 1946, 1948 and 1952).

Origins of the Thrombogenic Theory

Unfortunately the description of the class-room episode published in 1946 gave the impression that the thrombogenic theory was the outcome of a technical error which, in fact, was not the case. The idea that intimal thickenings must be thrombotic had been gradually dawning over the years and was the logical outcome of the conviction that the overgrowth theory must be wrong. Clearly,

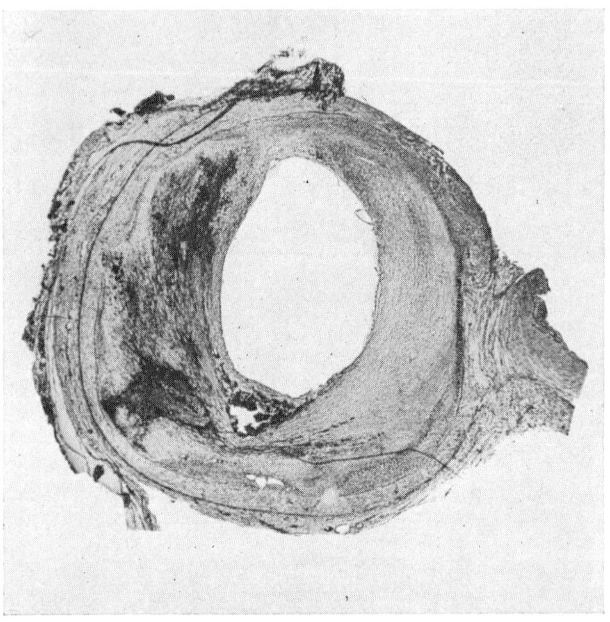

FIG. 5. Coronary atherosclerosis. Section from the same artery as shown in fig 4 but from a point about 4 mm distant from that section. The two channels have joined to form a single lumen and the thrombus is now a fibrous thickening of the intima which, being fatty, constitutes atherosclerosis. Frozen section: Sudan III and haemalum, $\times 20$.

the most likely way by which the lumen of a pulsating artery could be reduced, apart from external compression, would be by something occupying it, such as a thrombus or embolus, but in the 1930s it would have been fruitless, merely on theoretical grounds, to suggest that this had any bearing on atherosclerosis. What was needed, and what the class-room episode at long last provided, was a way of showing beyond reasonable argument that intimal thickenings could be thrombotic, and that the concept was not purely imaginary.

The concept was in fact not new. Ziegler, in his textbook of 1896–97 mentions fibrin thrombi in the arteries forming thickenings like those of endocarditis, and Mallory (1912–13) refers to the organisation of fibrin as a common source of intimal thickening. More recent observers including Clark, Graef and Chasis (1936), Boyd (1938) and Horn and Finklestein (1940) noted the incorporation of mural thrombi into the arterial walls, but none of them specifically related the process to atherosclerosis. Undoubtedly Mallory must have had it in mind, however, when he wrote: 'The elevated plaques of fibrous tissue on the intimal surface of the aorta are usually, perhaps always formed in that way'. He was evidently not prepared to take issue against the long accepted growth theory, but his 'perhaps always' seems to denote more than a slight leaning in that direction. The fibrin deposit idea must have been in the minds of pathologists for years but it was too unorthodox for current teaching.

Rokitansky

The thrombogenic theory in fact originated long before the present century. In Carl v. Rokitansky's Manual of Pathological Anatomy, translated by George M. Day (1852), there was the following account of atheroma:

'*Excessive deposition on the lining membrane of the vessels* . . . In a highly developed form of this affection, we find the inner surface of a large artery, as the aorta, covered with a foreign substance spread over it at separate points, or in large patches and forming a stratum varying in thickness, by which the inner surface of the vessel is commonly rendered uneven. . . . It varies in thickness . . . and extends in extreme cases over the whole trunk and main branches of the aorta, implicating the entire arterial system.

The deposition is generally the thickest directly over the division of a trunk, or at the bifurcation of a vessel. At these points the deposit is frequently so thick, that the mouths of the divergent vessels are much contracted, and even wholly closed. . . .

At its commencement, this deposition cannot be detected without a previous familiarity with its appearance. It is then a delicate, soft, succulent membrane, exhibiting a vitreous transparency. . . .

The deposition continually increases in thickness by the addition of new strata, and thus gradually passes from the condition of transparency and succulence, characteristic of recent formations, to the state in which it appears opaque, resembling coagulated albumen, and finally presents a ligamentous appearance, having a dull, wrinkled surface.

The atheromatous process consists in the metamorphosis (disintegration) of the deposit, into a pulpy mass, compared by the French to a purée of peas, consisting of large crystals of cholesterin, fatty globules, and of molecules exhibiting various degrees of consistence, from coarseness to extreme fineness, and consisting of albumen and calcareous salts.'

Rokitansky summarises his views as follows:

'The deposit cannot be regarded as a product (exudation) of an inflammaticn in the arteries . . . The deposit is an exogenous product derived from the blood, and for the most part from the fibrin of the arterial blood. Its formation demonstrates the pre-existence of a peculiar crasis of the blood, which is intrinsically *arterial,* although at the present time we are wholly ignorant of the peculiarity on which it depends'.

It must seem surprising that Rokitansky's teaching played no part in the development of the modern thrombogenic theory, but it should be explained that in the present century his views on atheroma were forgotten and his name was no longer associated with the subject. Modern pathology, we were taught, began with Virchow, and most writings dating from before his were considered to be of no more than historical interest. Virchow (1856) rejected Rokitansky's interpretation of atheroma on histological grounds, arguing that the changes were subendothelial and not surface deposits, and such was Virchow's influence that the thrombogenic theory was dismissed and forgotten, even Rokitansky himself having apparently abandoned it.

Confirmation

Soon after the reintroduction of the thrombogenic theory in 1946 support for it came from Harrison (1948) when he showed that fibrous thickenings of the pulmonary arteries could be produced in rabbits by injecting fibrin particles into their veins. The particles lodged in the pulmonary arteries (fig 6) and were in due course covered with endothelium (fig 7) and incorporated into the vessel walls (fig 8) where they formed fibrous plaques (fig 9). His experiments were repeated with similar results by Heard (1952) and later by Professor Egon Lichtenberger, to whom the writer is indebted for the accompanying illustrations, (figs 6–9). More

FIGS 6–9. Experimental pulmonary embolism. Fibrin particles injected into veins of rabbits on three successive days are lodged in pulmonary arteries and converted into intimal thickenings. All are paraffin sections, haemalum and eosin, ×20.
(I am much indebted to Professor Egon Lichtenberger for these illustrations.)

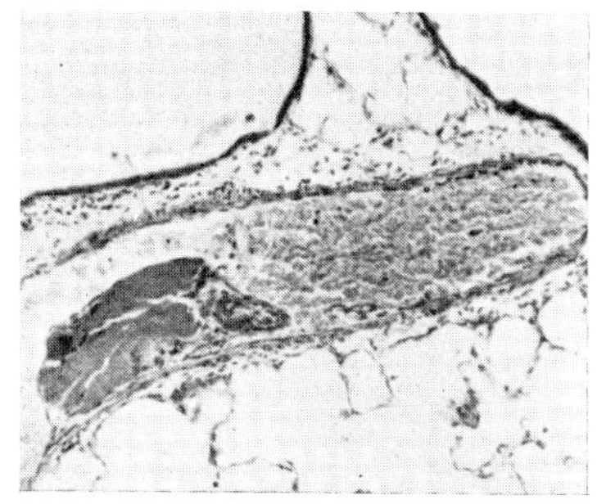

FIG. 6. On 4th day after first injection. The fragment of fibrin is attached to the vessel wall and partly covered with endothelium.

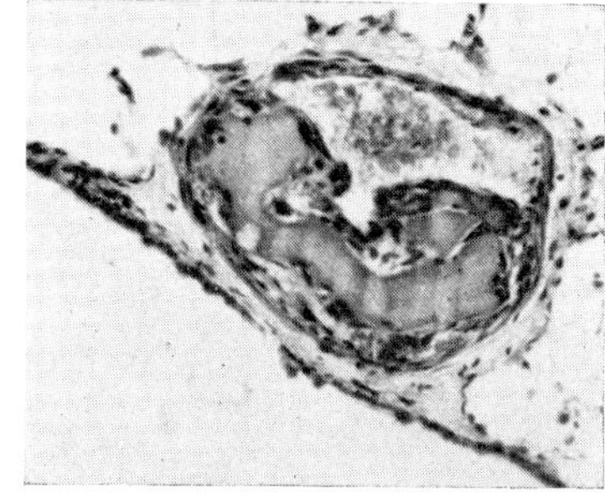

FIG. 7. On 6th day after first injection. A well defined layer of endothelium covers the fragment of fibrin which is now hyaline in appearance.

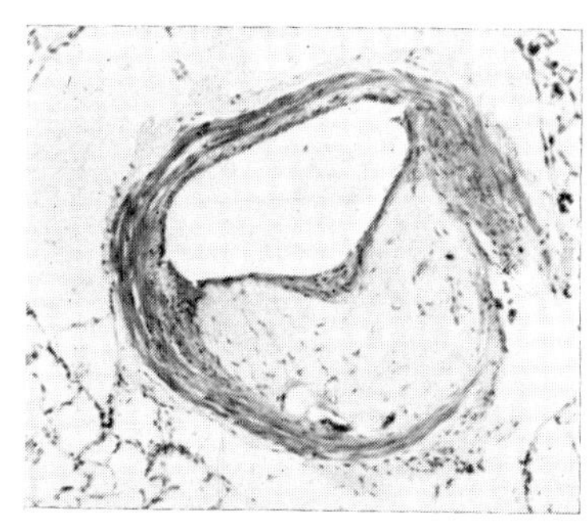

FIG. 8. After two months. A mass of hyaline substance is embedded in the intima and moulded to form a crescentic thickening.

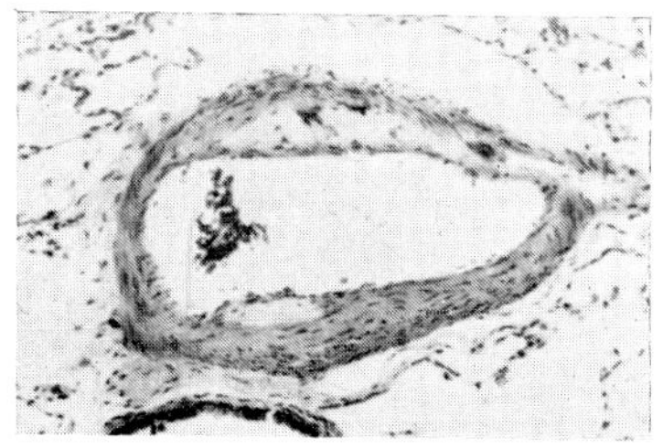

FIG. 9. After six months all that remain are fibrous thickenings of the intima.

recently Crawford and Woolf (1969) reported the production of atheroma-like lesions in pig aortas following the development of mural thrombi induced by gentle scarification of the intimal surface.

Supporting evidence was also forthcoming from studies of various human tissues, including the aorta by Geiringer (1951), McLetchie (1952) and Crawford and Levene (1952), renal arteries by Heard (1949), and especially the coronary arteries by Morgan (1956) to whose important work reference will again be made in a later chapter (p 48). Thus, it came to be fairly widely acknowledged that some, at least, of the thickenings in atherosclerosis were thrombotic in origin, and this was profoundly reassuring since it showed that the line of reasoning set out on pages 10 and 12, although contrary to current opinion, was not unsound, and might justifiably be carried further in the interpretation of arterial lesions.

Chapter Four

Arterial Thrombi

One may examine scores of aortas without seeing anything like thrombi as commonly represented, not because they are rare, but because in time they become so changed as to be almost unrecognisable, or recognisable only with experience.* To find easily identifiable thrombi one should study the coronary arteries from cases of fatal occlusion, where fresh fibrin is practically always to be found and where one can usually observe some of the changes it undergoes in its conversion to fibrous tissue.

Coronary Thrombi

In the coronary arteries thrombi of various sizes occur, ranging from large masses practically filling the lumina (fig 10) down to minute flakes of fibrin loosely attached to the intimal surface (fig 11). They are almost entirely confined to the extramyocardial vessels, and mostly located at flexures and bifurcations. Recently formed thrombi are usually found on the surfaces of older fibrous thickenings which are themselves products of thrombi and, on studying fatal cases, it soon becomes evident that coronary thrombosis tends to be a recurring condition with successive deposits forming one on top of another. If the thrombi are large and recur in rapid succession they produce cumulative thickenings which may result in progressive narrowing of the lumina until in the end it may require only a minute thrombus to bring about complete occlusion (fig 12). In most cases, however, the thrombi are not large enough to obstruct the arteries and, although they may cause considerable thickenings of the intima, the thickenings, by reducing the elasticity of the vessel walls, are more likely to lead to widening of the arteries than narrowing (see chap 7).

* It cannot be too strongly emphasised that, for the study of lesions in the larger arteries, frozen sections are of the greatest value, not only for the demonstration of fatty changes but also for the differentiation of the connective tissues. The heating and dehydration involved in paraffin embedding tend to shrink and fuse fibrin and connective tissues to such a degree that it is often difficult to distinguish them, whereas in frozen sections they are usually clearly distinguishable by their differences in refractility, even without staining. Likar *et al.* (1969) have also noted that microthrombi in bovine arteries are more easily detected in frozen sections than in paraffin ones.

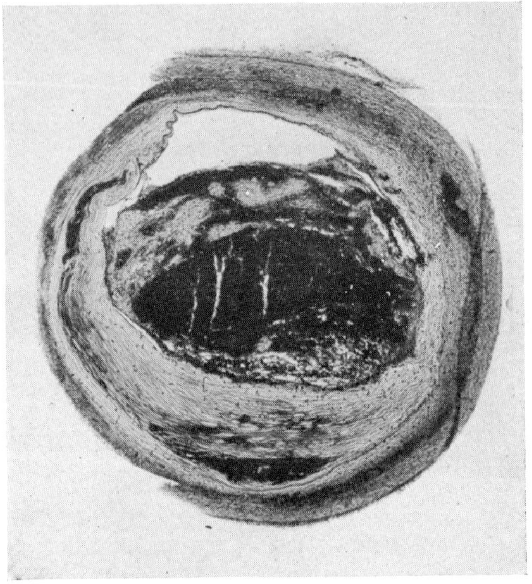

FIG. 10. Recent coronary thrombosis. The thrombus from its shape looks as if it had originally occluded the lumen and later retracted. It is mostly composed of fibrin but the black area is blood clot representing recent haemorrhage. In the vessel wall at the lower part there is an old atherosclerotic thickening.
Frozen section: Sudan III and haemalum, ×8.

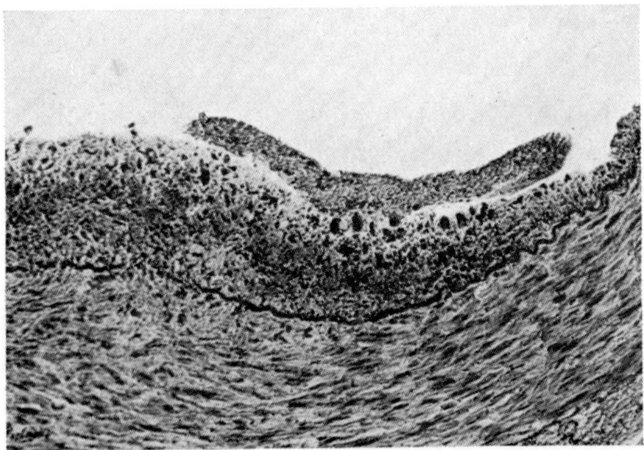

FIG. 11. Microthrombus in coronary artery. Recently formed thrombi of this kind are readily washed off at autopsy and are liable to be missed. Frozen section: Sudan III and haemalum, ×80.

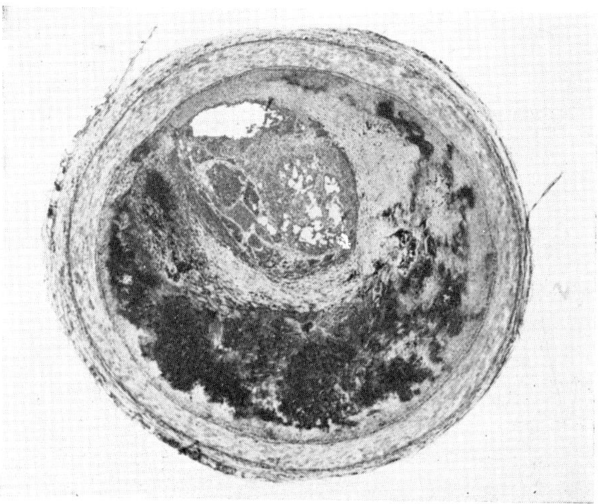

Fig. 12. Coronary atherosclerosis with terminal occlusion. A fibrous thickening with much fatty change, showing as black area, involves more or less the whole circumference of the vessel wall. The greatly reduced lumen is occupied by a terminal thrombus which originally caused total occlusion but part of which has been broken off and lost. Frozen section: Sudan III and haemalum, × 15.

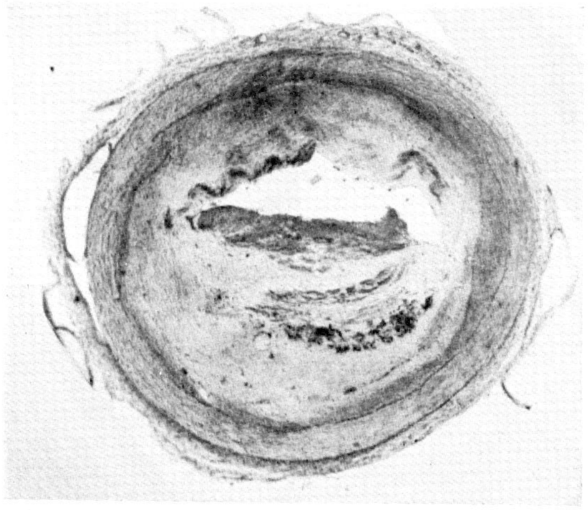

Fig. 13. Coronary atherosclerosis with recent mural thrombus. An old fibrous thickening with relatively little fatty change involves most of the vessel wall whilst a recent fibrin thrombus occupies much of the lumen. Frozen section: Sudan III and haemalum, × 15.

3

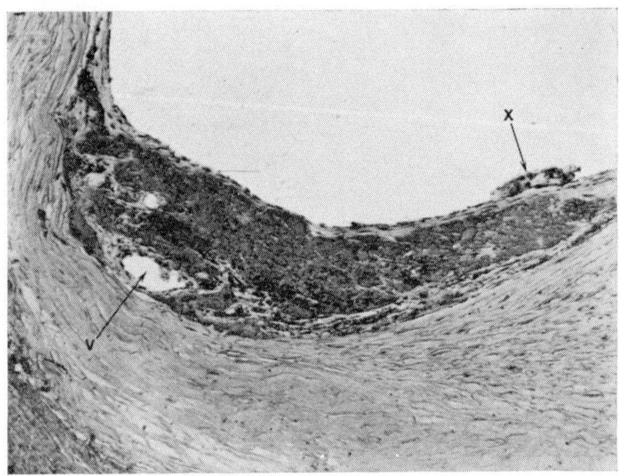

FIG. 14. Incorporation of mural thrombus. The dark mass consists of hyaline fibrin which is undergoing organisation with vascularisation in the deeper layers at v, and a sub-endothelial layer of clear fibrous tissue covering its surface. A microthrombus is seen on the surface at x. Frozen section: Sudan III and haemalum, ×60.

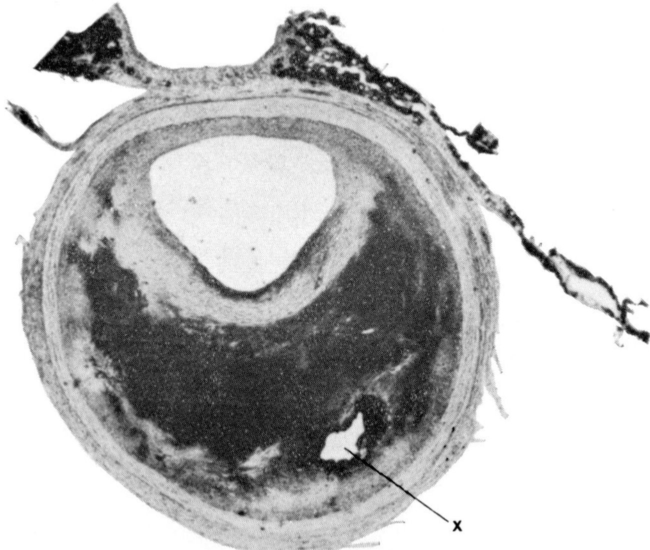

Fig. 15. Incorporation of mural thrombus. The thrombus is part of the intima and compressed to form a crescentic thickening comparable with that shown in fig. 8. There is much fatty change with a focus of calcification at x. Frozen section: Sudan III and haemalum, ×15.

Thrombi when newly formed usually stand out prominently and may be ragged (fig 13), but later they become smoothed out and covered with endothelium so that they are incorporated into the vessel walls (fig 14). At first they appear to be composed mainly of fibrin which, in frozen sections stains specifically with methyl violet but in time the fibrin becomes compressed into a more homogeneous, 'hyaline' substance which stains indifferently, making its identification more difficult. Later, under the influence of the blood flow, the thrombi are gradually flattened out and moulded to the shape of the vessel walls (fig 15) and, in due course, by a process of organisation they are converted into fibrous thickenings of the intima. But by this time the picture tends to be obscured by fatty changes.

Aortic Thrombi

Atherosclerosis is commonest in the aorta and it is to that vessel one should next turn to study the part played by thrombosis, but it must not be expected that recognisable thrombi will always be seen there. Most mural thrombi are too small to be easily seen, in fact most are microscopic, whilst even the larger ones tend to become so

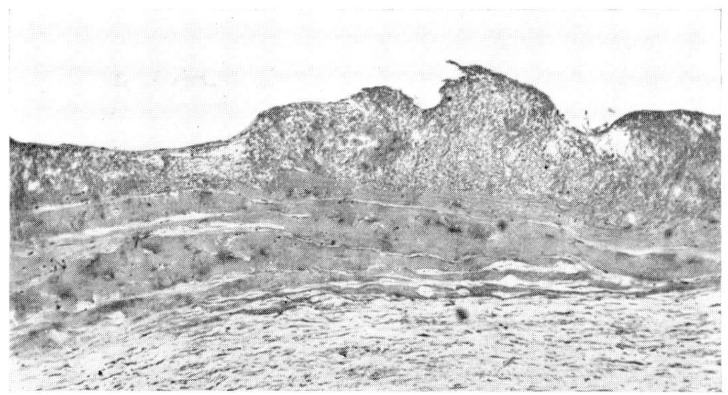

FIG. 16. Steps in transformation of mural thrombi. The surface layer is newly formed fibrin. Beneath it there are older condensed layers of hyaline fibrin alternating with thinner layers of clear fibrous tissue in which there are spindle shaped connective tissue cells. Towards the deeper parts the clear layers appear progressively thicker at the expense of the hyaline fibrin which is gradually replaced, and finally the fibrous tissue merges into that of the adjacent intima. Frozen section: Sudan III and haemalum, × 15.

quickly changed that they escape detection. To find easily identifiable thrombi one should study the abdominal aorta in elderly subjects where the severest lesions are to be seen, and where the intima is often thickly strewn with atheromatous plaques leaving little of its surface unaffected. There thrombosis is a recurring process, with multiple deposits one on top of another, forming strata of different ages (fig 16). In such examples the successive stages in the transformation of fibrin to fibrous tissue may be seen, with fresh layers of fibrin on the surface, older hyaline fibrin subjacent, or external to it, and still older, partly organised fibrin in the outer layers merging into the fibrous tissue of the surrounding intima.

Sometimes this sequence is upset by the fact that thin deposits are more quickly organised than thicker ones, with the result that substantial layers of hyaline substance, representing unorganised fibrin, may occasionally be found buried under thinner layers of fully organised fibrous tissue (fig 17), producing appearances which have been mistaken for degenerating connective tissue and cited as examples of a 'collagen degeneration'. How long it takes to convert fibrin to fibrous tissue is hard to estimate, but the fact that fresh fibrin is rarely seen suggests that the transformation process is not long delayed.

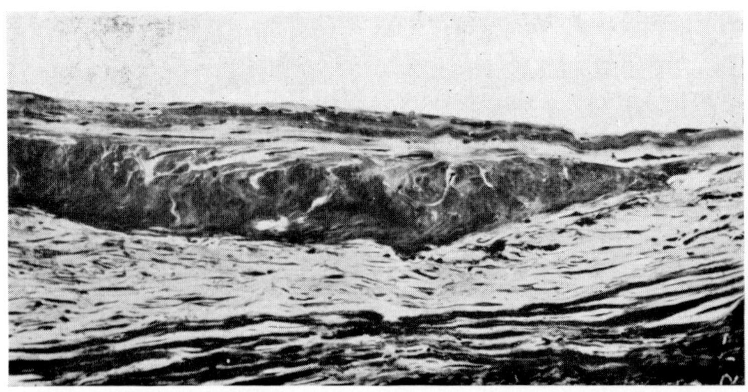

FIG. 17. Hyaline thrombus embedded in intima. The darker layers are hyaline fibrin and the paler ones newly formed fibrous tissue. The fibrous tissue is formed around spindle shaped connective tissue cells which appear to have invaded the fibrin. This is shown in the central dark layer which is hyaline fibrin in which there are early signs of invasion by connective tissue cells. Frozen section: Sudan III and haemalum, × 120.

Fine Encrustations or Microthrombi

In young subjects arterial thrombi are seldom conspicuous and have consequently been regarded as rare, but careful study shows that this is far from true. Most mural thrombi are, in fact, too small to be readily detectable by the naked eye at autopsy and, moreover, the recently formed ones are often so loosely attached to the vessel wall that they are liable to be detached and washed away in processing specimens for histology (fig 11). Most of them are microscopic (figs 2 and 18–22), and the term 'microthrombi' is probably the more appropriate.

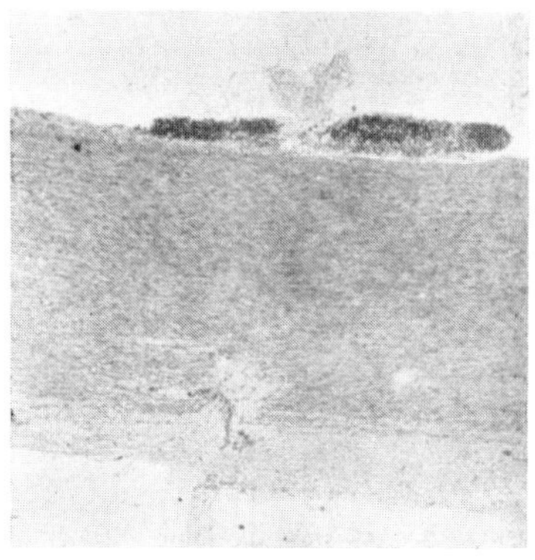

FIG. 18. Microthrombus in aorta of child aged three years who died of acute leukaemia. The deposit appears to consist mostly of leukaemic cells and fibrin. The subjacent intima shows no apparent pathological change. Frozen section: Sudan III and haemalum, × 15.

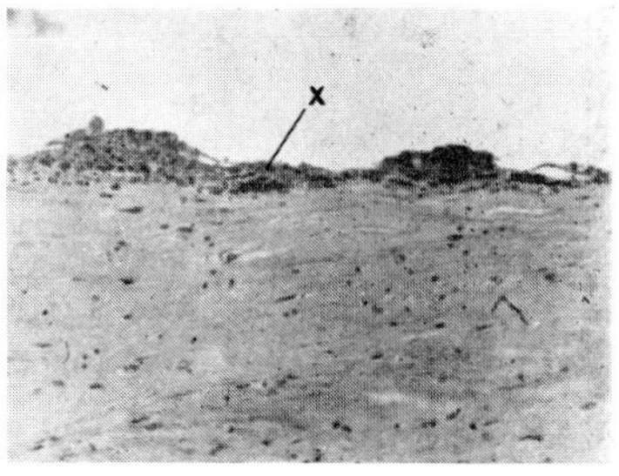

FIG. 19. Microthrombus on surface of atherosclerotic plaque. A fibrin deposit has been partly broken off leaving a ragged surface. The minute cluster of cells at x possibly represents an endothelial reaction to injury. Frozen section: Sudan III and haemalum, × 20.

Only occasionally in the past have the so-called fine encrustations been noted and, as a rule, they have not been represented as of much importance. Often they are chance findings but they can be detected with the aid of a hand lens as slight furrings of the intimal surface. Their frequency became apparent when an attempt was made to estimate the incidence of fresh fibrin deposits in arteries, and was found to be unexpectedly high. Taking aortas from unselected subjects of all ages, it was found that more than three times as many showed microthrombi as showed gross fibrin deposits and that in the positive examples microthrombi were immeasurably more

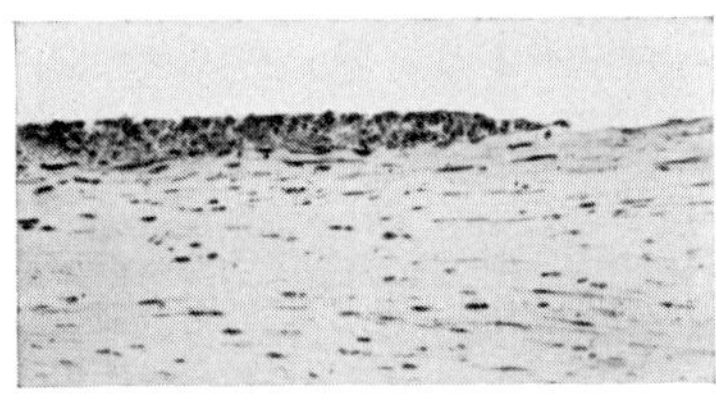

FIG. 20. The microthrombus is more finely granular than that shown in fig. 19 and probably consists largely of platelets. Frozen section: Sudan III and haemalum, ×75.

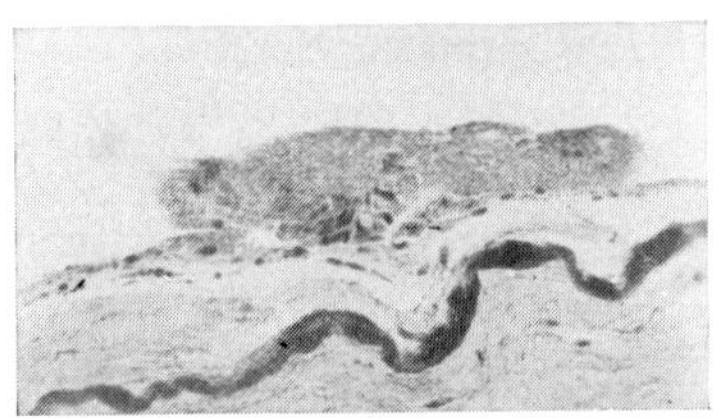

FIG. 21. A minute flake of fibrin is clearly associated with a cluster of swollen endothelial cells suggesting a reaction to injury. The dark wavy line in the intima is a buried layer of unorganised fibrin. Frozen section: Sudan III and haemalum, ×90.

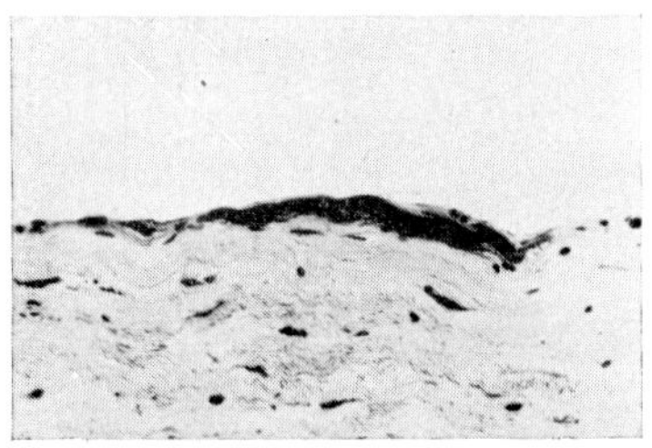

FIG. 22. Microthrombus incorporated into intima. This lesion which was found by chance was hardly visible even microscopically but was shown up by its refractility when viewed by oblique transillumination. Frozen section: Sudan III and haemalum, ×110.

numerous than larger deposits. Once familiar they were recognised with increasing frequency, not only in the aorta but in medium sized arteries including the coronaries (fig 11). Most of them were deposited on the surfaces of older organised thrombi, but some were found in the otherwise normal looking aortas of young children, that shown in fig 18, for example, being from the aorta of a child of three years who died from acute leukaemia. Another was found in the aorta of a boy of seven who had a cerebral tumour. The writer has not studied the arteries of lower animals in this connection but Likar and his co-workers have reported that they are common in bovine coronary arteries, remarking incidentally that they are more easily detected in frozen sections than in paraffin ones. Thus it is only in the last twenty or so years that we have come to realise how common fibrin deposits in arteries are and what a potential source of intimal thickening they must be in the course of a life-time.

Platelet Thrombi

The composition of microthrombi varies, some consisting mainly of fibrin (figs 11, 12 and 19) and others containing leucocytes and granular material (fig 20), which we assume to be mainly blood platelets. Unfortunately platelets are not easily identifiable in sections of human arteries, especially if the thrombi have developed some time before death, or if fixation of the tissues has been long delayed. Jørgensen *et al.* (1967) have observed that the composition of experimentally produced thrombi changes, consisting mainly of platelets at the outset but becoming predominently fibrinous after ten or eleven days. It is not surprising, therefore, that platelets have not in the past been generally recognised in studies of arterial lesions, and that it is only in recent years that their importance in the pathogenesis of atherosclerosis has come to be appreciated.

Information on the functions of the blood platelets has been summarised by French (1968 and 1971) and by Mustard and his co-workers (1968). From them we learn that when the endothelial lining of an artery is breached and circulating platelets come into contact with the collagen of the intima they adhere to it and, releasing adenosine diphosphate which increases their adhesiveness, they form aggregates covering the breach. They also release a clotting agent and become centres of fibrin formation which serves to bind them *in situ*. Thus, it may be inferred that the laying down of platelets and the formation of mural thrombi represent a repair process. Admittedly it is difficult to show definite evidence of this histologically, the endothelium being as a rule missing where a thrombus is attached to a vessel wall, and whether the loss of endothelium is cause or effect is difficult to determine. Only occasionally does one see anything like a cellular reaction as in fig 21 and even then the interpretation is difficult. It is also difficult to determine what become of microthrombi. Fibrin may be resolved leaving no trace but it is doubtful if platelets are so easily disposed of. Some microthrombi undoubtedly remain permanently and are incorporated into the intima (fig 22), so that they must be regarded as likely sources of intimal thickening. As will be explained in a later chapter, evidence is accumulating which suggests that microthrombi may be the commonest source of the intimal thickening that goes with ageing.

In recent years interest has been aroused by the finding (O'Brien (1968), Zucker and Peterson (1970) and others) that acetylsalicylic acid and other non-steroidal anti-inflammatory agents inhibit ADP-induced platelet aggregations *in vitro*. This may seem to offer some promise of a method of controlling arterial thrombosis, but in contemplating such remedies it must be borne in mind that not all thrombi are necessarily harmful (see Chap 11); platelet thrombi are probably mainly beneficial.

Chapter Five

Retrogressive Changes

Soon after they are formed arterial thrombi begin to undergo various changes by which they are more or less disguised, and it is these changes that account for most of the complex histological appearances seen in atherosclerosis.

Shrinkage and Softening

In the coronary arteries one not infrequently sees thrombi which, judging by their shape and position, must originally have occluded the lumina but later having shrunk, become partially detached from the vessel wall, and retracted, leaving lateral spaces for blood to pass (fig 10). Such spaces become lined with endothelium and form channels which, under the influence of the re-established blood pressure, are gradually enlarged, the thrombi being pushed aside and compressed against the vessel wall until in the end they are reduced to crescentic thickenings of the intima (fig 15). Although not generally recognised, this process, which may be said to be a form of canalisation, probably accounts for most of the survivals in cases of coronary occlusion.

Thus coronary occlusion is not necessarily an irreversible condition, and the sequence of events in coronary disease may be practically the reverse of what we have been led to imagine. Instead of an overgrowth of the intima gradually encroaching on the lumen and narrowing it, there is a sudden reduction or even total occlusion of the lumen followed by a gradual reopening of it as the thrombus shrinks. In this way an arrested circulation may be restored and it is not uncommon to find patent arteries leading to old myocardial infarcts making it look as if infarctions occurred without occlusion. On the other hand, most arterial thrombi are of the mural type but, as they tend to recur, successive deposits may build up so that narrowing becomes progressive. In that case, however, the progress is intermittent, and after each narrowing there is a gradual widening again as the thrombus shrinks. If further thrombosis can be prevented the widening may progress until the circulation is in a considerable measure restored.

Another change which may contribute to the reduction of a thrombus is softening, of which the most striking examples are seen in red thrombi. Erythrocytes, when no longer in circulation, disintegrate and, if they are present in large masses, their break-down leaves spaces filled with a semi-fluid fatty debris. These spaces may form permanent foci of fatty change resembling atheroma but, as will be explained later, they differ essentially from the true atheroma (p. 32).

Hyaline Change

This is perhaps the most controversial of the changes occurring in mural thrombi because it is the one by which they are most rapidly disguised. Most large mural thrombi are composed mainly of fibrin which in its early form is easily identifiable and stains specifically with methyl violet. Later it becomes compressed into a more or less homogeneous substance which Gitlin and Craig (1957) and Lendrum *et al.* (1962) have shown to be variable in its staining reactions. It then bears no resemblance to fresh fibrin, but is described as 'hyaline' (figs 16 and 17) or, if it has not entirely lost its specific staining properties, as 'fibrinoid', and is sometimes taken for degenerate collagen. Levene (1955) has confirmed by electron-microscopy that the material in atherosclerosis having the appearance of hyaline collagen consists largely of fibrin, and this has been confirmed by Still and Boult (1957). Electron-microscopy, however, is not entirely conclusive because, whilst it may confirm the presence of fibrin in the material in question, it cannot confirm that the material is entirely fibrin, and the same applies to the fluorescent antibody method of identification. In fact, the strongest evidence that the hyaline material is altered fibrin is, after all, in the histological picture as shown in fig 16, where the material in question occupies an intermediate position in what is clearly a transition from fibrin to fibrous tissue.

Fatty Changes

The fatty changes in arterial lesions are usually considered as representing a single process, whereas there are at least three categories of fatty change differing not only in their appearance and distribution but also in their mode of development. Although they are not all products of thrombosis, it will be convenient to consider them all under the present heading so that they can be more readily compared and distinguished.

1 *Fatty Changes in Thrombi*

Most mural thrombi develop some fatty changes but in fibrin thrombi they are usually slight, consisting of no more than thin sprinklings of minute lipid droplets which, with Sudan III gives what looks like a faint yellow dusting of the fibrin layers. When the thrombi are eventually organised the fats mostly disappear leaving only a few droplets in the occasional macrophages which may be scattered about the region. In red thrombi the fatty changes are usually much more plentiful, the solid masses of erythrocytes and other cells breaking down and forming softenings containing mixtures of neutral fats, fatty acids and cholesterol. At one time it seemed to the writer that atheroma might be entirely accounted for by this process, i.e. by a metamorphosis of the thrombi as Rokitansky suggested, but that idea soon had to be abandoned because even in the reddest of thrombi there was seldom so much fatty material as is seen in the average atherosclerotic plaque.

2 *Fatty Streaking*

This debatable lesion is most characteristically seen in the aortas of young subjects who have died from acute febrile conditions. It consists of minute clusters of lipophages lying immediately under the endothelium and forming slightly raised yellowish streaks, mostly on the posterior wall of the aorta, between the openings of the intercostal arteries. The streaks are usually finely beaded and run in the long axis of the vessel. Microscopically one sees in addition to the surface clusters, stray lipophages in the depth of the intima and sometimes the tissues around the internal elastic lamina are thinly dusted with minute lipid droplets. In the thin sections commonly used in histology the lipophages are often too widely dispersed microscopically to appear very numerous but, as Zinserling (1925) and Holman and his co-workers (1958) have shown, when the aorta is stained in bulk with Sudan, they are often plentiful enough in depth to colour the intima a bright orange.

Some observers regard fatty streaking as an early stage of athero-sclerosis but others disagree on the grounds that the two lesions do not always coincide in distribution. One tends to think of lipophages as wandering cells, possibly acting as scavengers, but in what direction they are wandering is difficult to conjecture. Rannie (1956) has suggested that there is a clearing process whereby substances which the body cannot metabolise are carried out through the arterial walls by macrophages, and certainly something like this is seen in the pulmonary arteries, but it is not easy to understand the relationship of this to atherosclerosis.

3 *Fatty Changes in Foci of Disruption – True Atheroma*

As pointed out on page 8, fatty debris occupies the spaces formed by the splitting apart of the layers resulting from stiffening of the intima (fig 3). These spaces are usually located in the outer layers

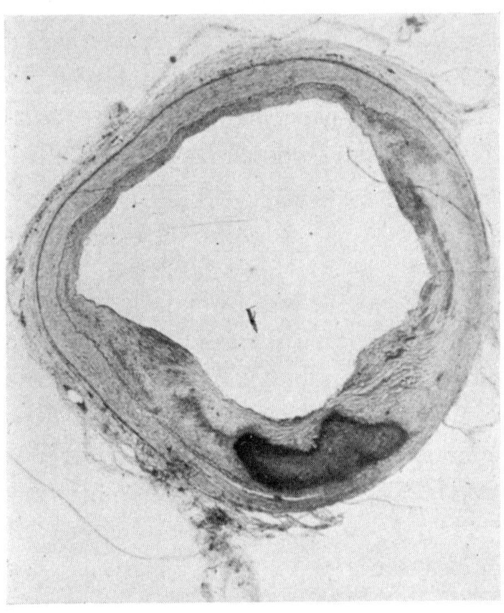

FIG. 23. Calcification in coronary artery. The dark patch in the lower part of the section is a calcified focus in an atherosclerotic thickening of the intima. It will be noted that the media adjacent to the thickening is thinned and the lumen is, if anything, widened. Frozen section: Sudan III and haemalum, ×20.

of the intima or between the intima and media (fig 25), and the fats in them are usually much richer in doubly refracting lipids than are the fatty deposits of category 1 which occur in the superficial layers of the intima and which are derived from the mural thrombi themselves.

In 1938 Winternitz, Thomas and LeCompte suggested that the fats in atheroma were derived from haemorrhage, and our findings entirely bear this out. As will be shown in chapter 8, with the splitting apart of the layers of the intima, blood is shed into the spaces and the eventual breakdown of its constituents yields haemosiderin and fatty debris. This, in the opinion of the present writer, is the true atheroma.

Calcification

Although not an essential part of atherosclerosis, calcified foci occasionally appear amongst atheromatous debris (fig 23), especially in elderly subjects. As Montgomery remarked, it seemed to be commoner in former years than now, or at least, it figured more prominently in older records than in the modern ones. This may be partly because older records were often based more on the gross findings at autopsy than on histological appearances. Calcareous foci are often of stony hardness so that they tend to be readily palpable at autopsy but attempts to cut through them usually result in tearing to pieces of the tissues. On gross examination therefore affected arteries give an impression of extremely destructive lesions but on histological examination after decalcification they are usually found to be widely patent (fig 23), without any suggestion of vascular impairment. Consequently, less importance is now attached to calcification in the coronary arteries than formerly.

Chapter Six

Progressive Changes

It is now fairly generally acknowledged that mural thrombi are converted into fibrous thickenings of the intima and, if one studies the histopathology of atherosclerosis with that process in mind, most of the changes are readily understandable.

Endothelialisation

Organisation probably begins almost immediately after a thrombus has formed, the first step being endothelialisation. Williams (1955) produced mural thrombi in the central arteries of rabbit's ears by local injury and noted coverings of endothelial cells forming in twenty-four hours. Crawford and Woolf (1968) produced mural thrombi on a larger scale in pig's aortas and observed endothelialisation on the third day.

In the past it has been assumed that the process is carried out by a growth of cells spreading from a neighbouring endothelial surface, but doubts have been cast on this by surgeons who have practiced arterial grafting. They have observed endothelialisation of large surfaces so far removed from any established endothelium that direct spread seemed unlikely, and this suggests the possible existence of other sources of cells with endothelialising potentialities such as the circulating blood. Ghani and Tibbs (1962) and Still and Ghani (1967), in carefully controlled experiments involving the implantation of plastic grafts into dog's aortas, have shown that such properties are possessed by cells which they identify as blood monocytes. Crawford and Woolf (1968) have suggested that the indigenous cells of thrombi have endothelialising potentialities, and a similar idea was implied by Dible (1966) when he described the formation of endothelial lined lacunae in the substance of thrombi at parts histologically far removed from any established endothelium. Recent support for this has been afforded by Davies, Ballantine, Robertson and Woolf (1975).

Vascularisation

Microthrombi appear to be converted into fibrous thickenings of the intima simply by the action of endothelial cells, but it would seem that when mural thrombi exceed a certain thickness

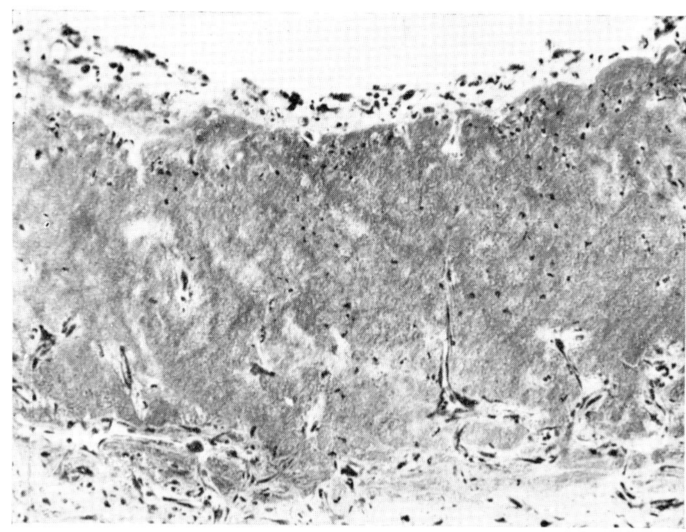

FIG. 24. Part of mural thrombus in aorta showing early vascularisation. The capillaries are entering mainly from the underlying intima. It will be noted that various blood leucocytes are included in the thrombus having presumably been enmeshed in the fibrin at its formation. Frozen section: Sudan III and haemalum, × 110.

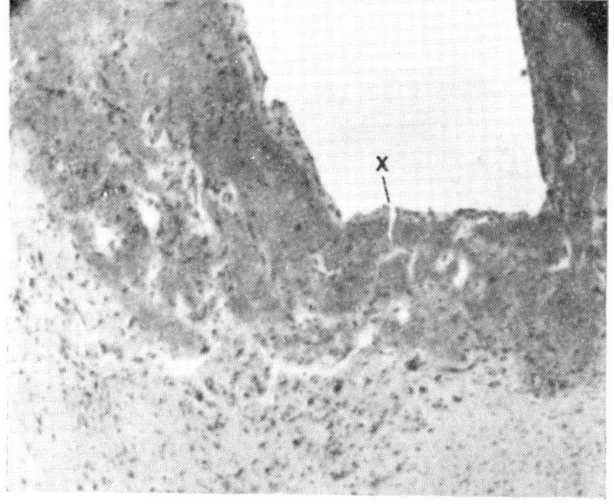

FIG. 25. Part of mural thrombus in coronary artery showing vascularisation. A capillary is seen entering from the lumen at x. Various cells are seen in the thrombus, some of them indigenous and some of them invading connective tissue cells. Frozen section: Sudan III and haemalum, × 80.

organisation calls for an augmented blood supply and, as Geiringer (1951), McLetchie (1952) and others have shown, this is provided by capillaries entering either from the intima (fig 24) or from the lumen of the artery (fig 25). From these sites vessels ramify to all parts so that for a time the thrombi are relatively vascular but later, when organisation is completed, most of the capillaries disappear. Those that remain are important as possible sources of haemorrhage which, as will be shown, is a factor in atherosclerosis.

Fibrous Tissue Formation

The cellular changes which go with organisation are familiar enough but it is still far from clear how a thrombus is changed into a fibrous thickening, whether by a direct transformation of the fibrin into collagen or by a resolution of the fibrin and a laying down of collagen in its place. Unfortunately, arterial studies have tended to confuse this issue by introducing hyaline change as an intermediate step with the result that we now have one and the same picture interpreted by one set of observers as fibrin undergoing hyaline change and by another as collagen undergoing 'fibrinoid' change. One thing seems clear, namely that cells play a determining part in the process, it being around certain spindle cells which lie between the layers of hyaline fibrin (figs 16 and 17) that the change occurs. Around each cell a zone of clearing forms in the hyaline material and gradually expands until neighbouring zones coalesce, and the whole mass is eventually converted into clearer collagenous tissue.

Some of the cells in this process are fibroblasts, or possibly smooth muscle cells, which have come in with the capillaries in vascularisation, but some are indigenous cells of the thrombi. Arterial thrombi are practically never without cells (figs 24 and 25). When newly formed they have the various leucocytes of the blood enmeshed in their fibrin and, although most of these in time disappear, some cells, probably the monocytes, remain and it seems likely that they become connective tissue-forming cells. In favour of this view is the fact that they are usually distributed through the substance of the thrombi in a way that suggests indigenous elements of the blood rather than invaders. The idea that fibroblasts may be derived from blood cells has for long been in the minds of pathologists, and has been discussed by Williams (1955) and by Ghani (1969).

Canalisation

It will have been noted that there are two ways in which the circulation through a thrombotic occlusion in an artery may be restored: (1) by the formation of new channels running through the thrombus as in fig 4, or (2) by partial detachment of the thrombus from the vessel wall and retraction, leaving a lateral space for blood to pass as in fig 10. The former is generally thought of as the classical canalisation and in connection with it there is the question as to how the channels are formed. It used to be thought that they were derived from the capillaries which took part in organisation, but Dible's suggestion that they are developed in the 'lacunae' which form in thrombi, probably by the action of fibrinolysin, seems more likely. At best, however, the classical canalisation must be a slow process and of little use in emergency.

By far the more important is the second way which involves retraction or shrinkage of the thrombus as explained on page 29. A lateral space or spaces are formed which become lined with endothelium and form new channels through which the blood flow is re-established. When blood pressure again comes into play one of the channels enlarges progressively and forms a new lumen, so that the circulation is more or less restored. Although not generally recognised this process must be one of the most important we have to consider, since it is the one which makes survival possible after coronary occlusion.

But the process is possible only if the tension in the vessel wall is low enough to allow relaxation and provided the wall is left free to stretch, as will be appreciated on comparing figs 10 and 12. In the artery shown in fig 10 there is still a considerable segment of the wall in which there is very little intimal thickening, so that stretching is still possible, whereas in fig 12 the intima around the whole circumference is so thickened by fibrous tissue that hardly any of it is left free to stretch, and consequently the very small thrombus in the lumen caused fatal occlusion. Thus, it is practically always in arteries already extensively thickened by previous thrombosis that fatal occlusion occurs. The writer has in fact never seen a case in which appearances indicated that a first coronory thrombosis was fatal. It is true that many individuals die in their first heart attack, but post-mortem examination in these cases always reveals older lesions of thrombotic type, usually with severe narrowing, having developed without the individual being aware of it, as was apparently the case in the artery shown in fig 39. There is, in fact, every indication that 'silent' coronary thrombosis is commoner than is generally supposed.

Elastosis

It was at one time thought that the presence of elastic fibres in intimal thickenings contraindicated an origin in thrombosis, but this was shown to be wrong when Harrison (1948) reported the development of elastic fibres in the thickenings produced in the pulmonary arteries of rabbits by injecting fibrin particles into their veins (p 17). Pathologists have been slow to acknowledge new formations of elastic tissue in arterial lesions, preferring to think of splitting of existing fibres rather than the development of new ones. Splitting of the internal elastic lamina used to be cited as an early sign of atheroma but views have changed and new formations of elastic fibres are now recognised. Dible (1966) has drawn attention to the striking increase of elastic fibres in the leg arteries with ageing, and appearances suggest that the same occurs, although perhaps to a lesser extent, in upper regions of the body.

Chapter Seven

Effects of Arterial Thrombosis

Anyone who has examined atherosclerotic arteries in the autopsy room knows how stiff the fibrous thickenings usually are, and will appreciate how they must interfere with movements and lead to disruption in pulsating arteries such as the aorta. In fact, they affect the arteries in different ways depending on their size relative to the vessels they occupy. If large they reduce the lumina simply by occupying them, but if not so large they may increase the lumina. To understand this paradox one must recall that it is their elasticity that enables the arteries to maintain their even mean diameters, and any loss of it lays them open to progressive stretching and dilatation.

Widening of Arteries

Mural thrombi, or the fibrous thickenings into which they are transformed, are less flexible or resilient than the normal vessel walls, and when firmly attached to these they tend to impede movements, especially contractions which depend on resilience. The affected segments are then clamped in the more or less expanded positions so that the media is stretched thin (figs 8 and 26). Medial thinning is usually most marked where the intimal thickening is abruptly localised, but the same effect is produced on a wider, though less conspicuous scale where intimal thickenings are more generalised, as in old age for example (chap 10). Then the change, although less accentuated, may involve the whole circumference of the vessel more or less (fig 38), with pronounced widening of the lumen, and this occurs not only in the aorta and its immediate branches but may extend far into the peripheral arteries in general, producing what Aschoff (1938) called the 'senile ectasis'.

In the peripheral arteries pulsation is less pronounced and discord therefore less in evidence, so that instead of focal disruption and fatty change, there is usually diffuse fibrous thickening with hardening of the vessel walls. This condition, which is referred to as 'diffuse arteriosclerosis', is practically universal in old age and, although it may not at first be very conspicuous, it involves stretching of the vessel walls in all directions, including lengthening as well as widening, with the result that in old age it becomes apparent in the familiar tortuosity of superficial arteries such as the temporals.

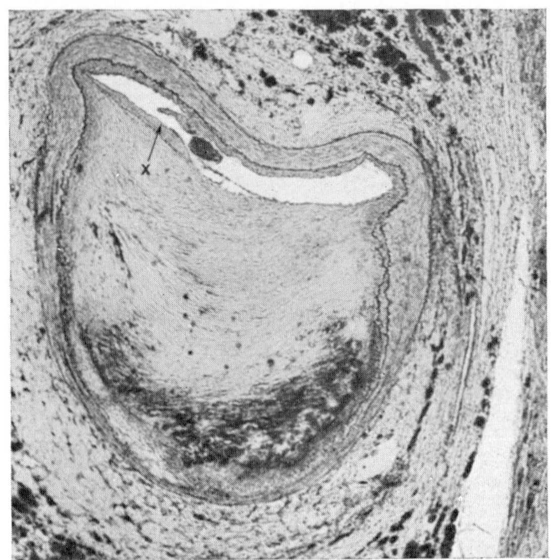

FIG. 26. Atrophy of media. The coronary artery shows a large mass of fibrous tissue occupying a bulge in the vessel wall. The appearance suggests an aneurysm but it is uncertain whether the outwards bulge or the fibrous mass in the lumen is the primary change. The mass is laminated with a recent deposit on its surface at x, suggesting that it has been formed gradually by successive deposits. It is notable that in spite of the large mass the lumen of the artery is not appreciably reduced. Frozen section: Sudan III and haemalum, ×25.

Infective Aortitis

While discussing dilatation of arteries it may be of interest to digress a little at this point to consider a condition in which the effects of loss of elasticity is especially well illustrated, namely syphilitic aortitis. In this now rather rare condition all three coats of the thoracic aorta are extensively infiltrated by a specific inflammatory process which destroys large patches of the medial muscle. In parts the whole thickness of the media is replaced by a granulation tissue which has little or no resilience, with the result that the full impact of the ventricular output bears on a tissue which is unable to yield and recoil like the normal vessel wall. The affected part then becomes progressively stretched and the end result is usually aneurysm formation and rupture.

Incidentally, the most prominent feature of syphilitic aortitis is fibrous thickening of the intima with fatty change or, in other words, atheroma, and it was not until about the end of last century that syphilitic aortitis was definitely recognised as distinct from atheroma. In syphilis the inflammation of the vessel wall promotes mural thrombosis on a scale never otherwise seen in the thoracic aorta and, in the active stage of the disease, the intimal surface is often smeared with blood and fibrin to such an extent that one wonders if perhaps it was in the study of cases of syphilitic aortitis that the thrombogenic hypothesis was first conceived.

Narrowing of Arteries

In the aorta mural thrombi are seldom large enough to reduce the lumen appreciably, but in medium sized arteries, such as the coronaries, even small thrombi may cause total occlusion. In studying such arteries it must, however, be remembered that they are usually in a state of post-mortem contraction, and their appearance must not be taken as a true representation of the state of affairs in life. There has undoubtedly been a tendency in the past to make this mistake and to classify as ischaemic such conditions as chronic interstitial myocarditis and nephrosclerosis on the grounds that the arteries supplying the affected parts appear narrowed, whereas the narrowing may be the effect rather than the cause of the condition.

When a mass of parenchyma is destroyed, from no matter what cause, there is usually a considerable reduction of its volume and of its capillary field so that it requires less blood and the arteries supplying it tend to close down, becoming thick walled and narrow like those of the involuting uterus. Yet it is notable that such arteries continue to supply enough blood for the tissues that remain. It would seem that, so long as arteries are patent, they are able to meet the needs of the tissues they serve and only when they are compressed or occluded by thrombi or emboli does ischaemia result.

Hard and Soft Atheroma

Atherosclerotic lesions vary in the amount of fatty material they contain depending, it would appear, on the balance of two inverse factors: the effects of pulse movements on mural thrombi, on the one hand, and the effects of mural thrombi on pulse movements on the other. In the aorta the majority of mural thrombi, or the fibrous thickenings into which they are transformed, are too small to have much effect on the movements of the vessel wall but, being them-

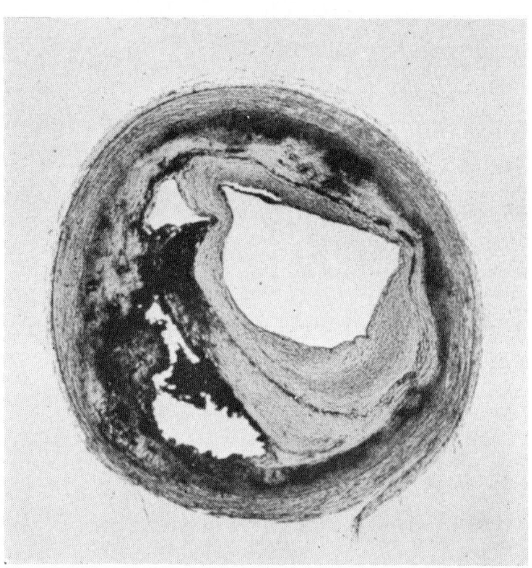

FIG. 27. Coronary artery showing the intense structural disorganisation which may be involved in atherosclerosis. The inner layers of the intima appear to consist of newly formed fibrous tissue and are widely separated from the outer layers by relatively large cavities containing fatty debris: an example of Montgomery's 'soft atheroma'. Frozen section: Sudan III and haemalum, ×20.

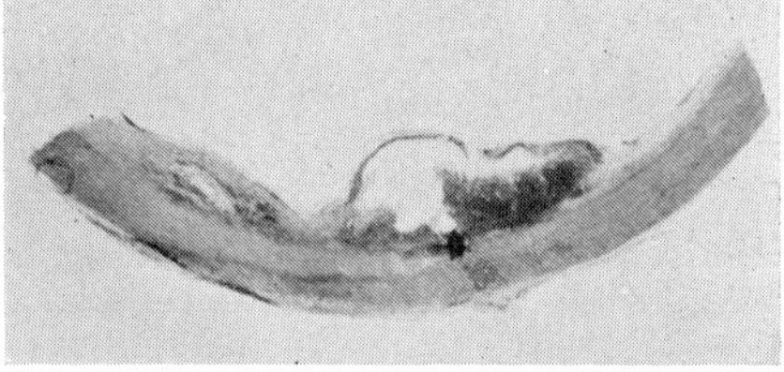

FIG. 28. In this example of Montgomery's soft atheroma in the aorta a thin layer of intima covers what was a relatively large accumulation of atheromatous debris most of which has been washed away. The layer is intact but rupture must have been imminent as the surrounding intima was extensively ulcerated. Frozen section: Sudan III and haemalum, ×4.

selves too stiff to comply with the movements, become crumpled and loosened in the way described on page 8 and shown in fig 3. Spaces are formed between the layers and these, being filled with fatty debris, constitute what Montgomery (1957–58) calls 'soft atheroma' (fig 27). Sometimes the spaces become distended with relatively large accumulations of fatty substance whilst the fibrous thickenings are relatively slight (fig 28), in which case the surface layers are liable to be torn away, leaving atheromatous ulcers which promote further thrombosis, and so the disease becomes progressive.

Large thrombi, on the other hand, may be firm enough or stiff enough to restrict movements, in which case disruption is reduced and, instead of prominent fatty deposits, lesions of a densely fibrous type (fig 2), sometimes called 'pearly plaques', or what Montgomery calls 'hard atheroma', are produced. Between Montgomery's hard and soft atheromas there is, of course, an infinite variety of intermediate types which, with the occasional addition of calcification, can account for all the complex histopathology of atherosclerosis.

Thus atherosclerosis is simply the disruption which must occur when a relatively unyielding mass of tissue is fixed to a structure which is constantly stretching and contracting.

Chapter Eight

Haemorrhage

The interpretations put forward in the foregoing chapters have all been based on the assumption that the larger arteries move in pulsation. That they do so cannot be doubted, but it may be questioned if pulse movements can ever be strong enough or extensive enough to tear the tissues in the way suggested. Most of the appearances studied are in some measure the effects of post-mortem contraction and it may therefore be suggested that they are all post-mortem effects. There is, however, evidence to refute this. In a high proportion of the lesions signs of old haemorrhage in the form of haemosiderin are present, indicating that the disruption has occurred some time before death.

Haemorrhage has long been recognised as an occasional finding in atherosclerosis but it has not as a rule been regarded as essential, and little attention was paid to it until Paterson (1936) noted its frequent occurrence in coronary lesions. Thereafter, interest was directed more to the question of its being a cause of coronary occlusion by compression of the lumen, than to the possible part it might play in the development of the lesions. In 1939 Winternitz, Thomas and LeCompte drew attention to haemorrhages in aortic atheroma, noting especially their frequency at the margins of the lesions, and these workers made the revolutionary suggestion that the haemorrhages were the source of the fatty changes in atheroma. They cited as a parallel example the haemorrhages in the degenerating colloid goitre which result in fatty changes rich in cholesterol and practically identical with atheroma. If their suggestion is right, and the evidence is strongly in its favour, the current views on the pathogenesis of atherosclerosis will have to be radically changed.

Haemosiderin

Extravasated blood soon disintegrates and decomposing corpuscles become unrecognisable, with the result that most atherosclerotic lesions examined in the laboratory show no signs of haemorrhage and offer no apparent evidence that haemorrhage is a factor in the lesions. A new light, however, was shed on this aspect of the problem when Paterson, Moffatt and Mills (1956) showed that, if unfixed aortas were immersed in a Prussian blue reagent, signs of old

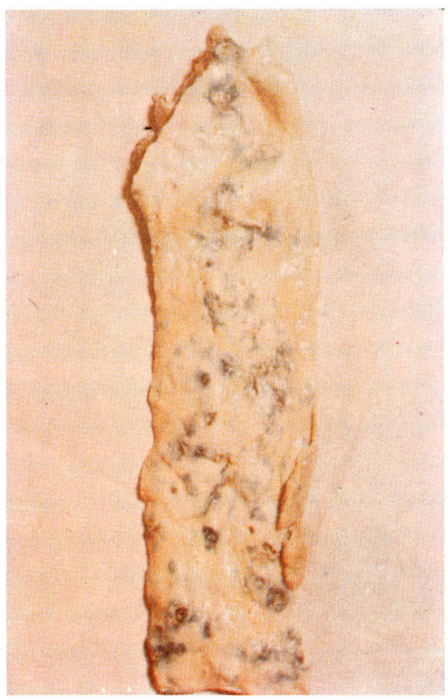

FIG. 29. Section of unfixed aorta which has been immersed overnight in Paterson's reagent. It shows the blue staining of haemosiderin in and around many of the atherosclerotic lesions.

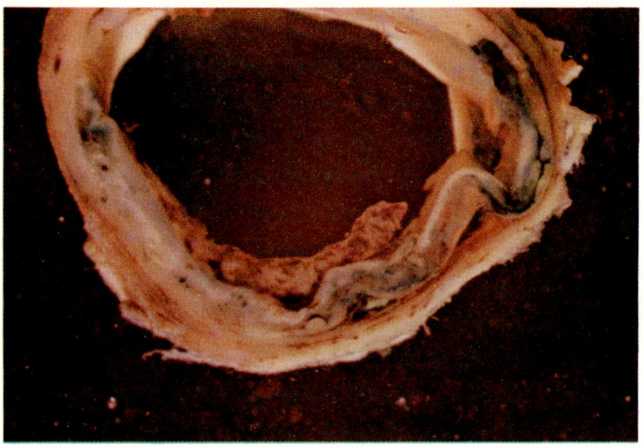

FIG. 30. Cross section of abdominal aorta following over-night immersion in Paterson's reagent. The crumpling effect of post-mortem contraction is shown with both freshly shed blood and blue stained haemosiderin associated with the splitting of the layers.

haemorrhage in the form of haemosiderin were seen in a high proportion of atherosclerotic lesions (fig 29). This seemed to offer a prospect of fresh information on the nature of arterial lesions and, in collaboration first with Dr R B Robertson (Duguid and Robertson, 1957) and later with Dr I Rannie (Rannie and Duguid, 1958), studies of the incidence of haemosiderin deposits in aortic lesions were undertaken by the writer.

Method

It seems that fixation in formalin or other watery solution tends to remove haemosiderin from the tissues and therefore unfixed arteries were used in this investigation. Sections of the vessels were obtained fresh at autopsy and immersed overnight in about ten times their volume of Paterson's reagent, a freshly prepared mixture of equal parts of potassium ferrocyanide (10 per cent) and hydrochloric acid (20 per cent). Next day, after washing in running water for two or three minutes, they were frozen and sliced across so as to provide smooth and even surfaces for viewing with reflected light. Since the blue staining of haemosiderin tends to fade if the preparations are mounted in a watery medium, permanent records were obtained by photography, the photographs (figs 30–34) being taken by flash-light with the specimens under water and using Ektachrome film. Strict precautions were not taken against exposure of the preparations to ferrous metals, but stainless steel knives and glass or plastic containers were used. It was found that any staining due to contamination was usually coarsely granular and confined to the surfaces of the sections, so that it was easily distinguishable from haemosiderin deposits which were always in the depths of the tissues.

Findings

We studied arteries from many regions and usually found some haemosiderin staining wherever there was atherosclerosis, but the one region time allowed us to study most systematically was the abdominal aorta. In a series of thirty-five consecutive autopsies, including subjects of various ages from six years and upwards, one whole cross section was taken from about an inch above the bifurcation and all but six of them, in fact all in which there was atherosclerosis, showed blue staining in a considerable proportion of the lesions. The arteries were not slit open lengthwise, so that in some of them the crumpling effects of post-mortem contraction were well shown, and the relationship of the haemosiderin to the disruption was obvious (fig 30). In some of the younger lesions

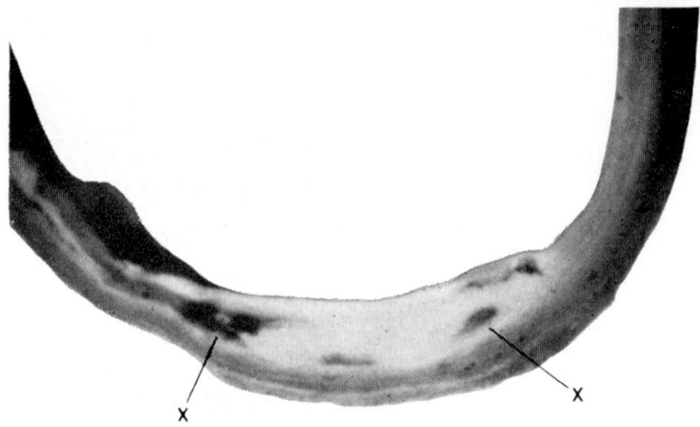

FIG. 31. Early atherosclerotic plaque from aorta of woman aged 38. The pale mass in the centre, consisting of fatty debris, is not clearly distinguishable from the surrounding tissues but immersion in Paterson's reagent has revealed small deposits of haemosiderin at each lateral margin (x) where the layers of the intima are being torn apart.

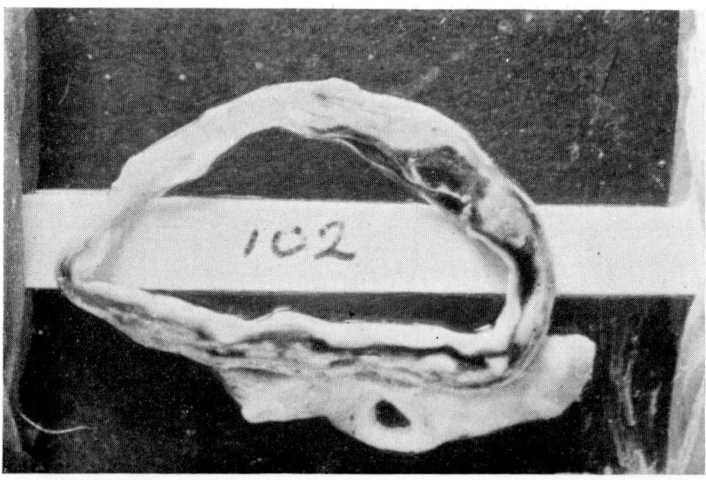

FIG. 32. Cross section of abdominal aorta from a women of 80 with advanced atherosclerosis. The wall is stretched thin and the lumen dilated. Treatment with Paterson's reagent shows haemosiderin tracking between the severed layers of the intima. Much fresh blood is present along with the haemosiderin.

the deposits were notably located at the margins of the plaques, just where the layers of the intima were being torn apart by the crumpling (fig 31), but in most of the preparations the haemosiderin was more extensive, tracking along the severed layers of the intima along with the fatty debris (fig 32) in which they were intimately mixed. Sometimes fresh haemorrhage was also present, especially at the margins of the lesions as Winterntiz *et al.* noted,

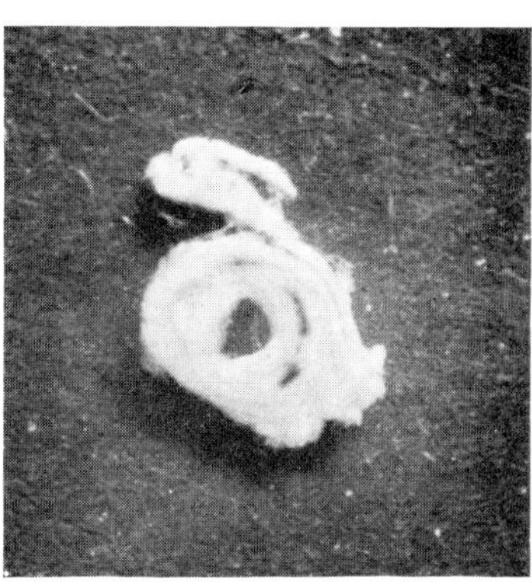

FIG. 33. Section of coronary artery showing several blue stained haemosiderin deposits in the thickened intima.

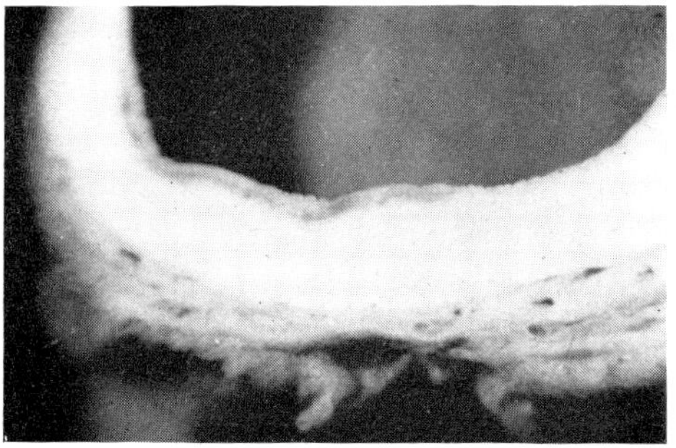

FIG. 34. Section of the wall of thoracic aorta from a girl aged 14 years. There is a subendothelial layer of blue stained haemosiderin which was associated with a patch of fatty streaking.

and in such cases blood, haemosiderin, fatty debris and cholesterol crystals were all mixed together in a way that seemed to denote a common source. Many coronary (fig 33) and other arteries were examined with similar results; wherever there was atheroma there were usually signs of haemosiderin. Several children's aortas with fatty streaking showed haemosiderin staining amongst the clusters of lipophages (fig 34) as Paterson and his colleagues noted.

Inference

It is acknowledged that haemosiderin deposits in tissues may be taken as representing old haemorrhage, and our findings therefore indicate that intimal haemorrhage occurs in life and is associated with the disruption of the tissues in atherosclerosis. Moreover, the closeness with which the haemosiderin coincides with the fatty changes seems strongly to indicate that the fats also are derived from old haemorrhage, as Winternitz *et al.* suggested. These findings came as no surprise to us as our previous observation that red thrombi are especially prone to fatty change had led us to think that erythrocytes were a source of the lipids. Other observers were of the same opinion: Morgan in his monograph on 'The Pathogenesis of Coronary Occlusion' (1956) expressed the opinion that repeated haemorrhages over long periods could well account for all the fatty accumulations in atherosclerosis, and it was his demonstration presented at the meeting of the Pathological Society of Great Britain and Ireland that finally convinced us of the relationship.

What did surprise us was the subsequent showing by Hand and Chandler (1962) that the blood platelets were a richer source of lipids than the erythrocytes. This was endorsed by Mitchell and Schwartz (1965) who reproduced figures published by Barkhan, Silver and O'Keefe (1961) showing that the total lipid content of erythrocytes amounts to only 1.26 per cent of dry weight, whereas that of platelets amounts to 17 per cent. Although platelets are smaller and less numerous than erythrocytes, it is still possible, in view of the apparent frequency with which intimal haemorrhage occurs that, over the years of a human life, they could well, as Morgan suggested, account for all the fatty accumulations we see in atherosclerosis. Probably the plasma lipids have also to be taken into account so that, as Rannie (1964) remarked, the amount and the type of the lipids in the lesions may reflect the amount and type of these in the plasma at the time of the haemorrhage.

Sources of Haemorrhage

Winternitz and his co-workers were interested in the vascularisation of the aortic intima and they were able to show that there were numerous small blood vessels from which haemorrhage could occur in atheroma. Later Paterson, Mills and Moffatt (1957) showed by the alkaline phosphatase method that capillaries are much more numerous in the aortic intima than they appear by ordinary staining methods. These capillaries may be sources of haemorrhage, but difficulty has been expressed in understanding how blood can leak from capillaries in which the pressure is comparatively low, into an intima which must be under a pressure equal to that of the blood in the lumen of the artery. This, however, need give rise to no difficulty because, whilst it is true that normally the tissues of the intima must always be under a positive pressure, the same may not always be true in pathological conditions. When the thickened intima is crumpled and the layers are torn apart, there must be phases in the pulse cycle when the pressures at the points of tearing are reduced and blood is actually sucked into the spaces. That blood gets into these spaces we know beyond question because it can be seen there, and that it disintegrates is shown by the fact that haemosiderin appears. Therefore it is only to be expected that other products of its destruction such as lipids would also appear and, whilst hemosiderin seems to be fairly readily absorbed, so that its presence in the lesions is transient, the lipids being less soluble remain and accumulate. Thus, we have reasonable answers to the two questions left over from chap 2 (p 10); we now know how the fibrous thickenings of the intima and the fatty changes are produced.

Chapter Nine

The Lipid Theory

To those who have learned to think of atherosclerosis as a disease of the lipid metabolism the suggestion that the fatty changes are simply products of haemorrhage may seem outrageous. The orthodox view that these changes are the cause of the disease is supported by a vast literature mostly of a clinical nature and outside the scope of this monograph, but the main basis of the lipid theory is experimental and rests on histological interpretations which may profitably be re-examined.

Origins of the Theory

Atheroma has long been ascribed to over-indulgence in food and drink, the idea no doubt arising from the fact that the aorta in obese subjects, who are generally supposed to have lived well, commonly shows much fatty change. In 1909, Ignatowsky, working on this hypothesis, succeeded in producing lesions like human atheroma in rabbits by feeding them on a protein-rich diet of milk, meat and eggs. Later Anitschkow and Chalatow (1913) showed that the lesions produced in this way were due, not to the protein, but to the cholesterol in the egg-yolk and they went on to show that the oral administration of pure cholesterol to rabbits resulted in atheroma-like deposits of this substance in their aortas. These experiments, which have been repeated countless times, are the basis of the lipid theory, and on the strength of them many believe that hyper-cholesterolaemia is the cause of atherosclerosis in man and further, that coronary disease is due to eating too much fat.

Not all authorities are agreed, however, that the administration of relatively enormous amounts of cholesterol to small herbivorous animals can have any bearing on the cause of disease in man, or that the lesions produced are truly comparable with human atherosclerosis. Since so much seems to depend on this question, Dr Rannie and the writer decided to review the experimental lesions in the light of recent information regarding the part played by thrombosis in the development of arterial lesions (Rannie and Duguid 1953).

Cholesterol Lesions

Twenty young, but fully grown rabbits were each given 1·5 g of crystalline cholesterol daily in their food and killed after periods ranging from five to forty-five weeks. All developed lesions in their aortas and some also in their pulmonary and other arteries, the lesions (e.g. fig 35) varying in numbers and severity depending on the length of time the respective animals had been under treatment. They were mainly scattered over the intimal surface of the thoracic aorta and consisted of heaped up deposits of cholesterol-bearing foam-cells, some of the deposits being covered with endothelium

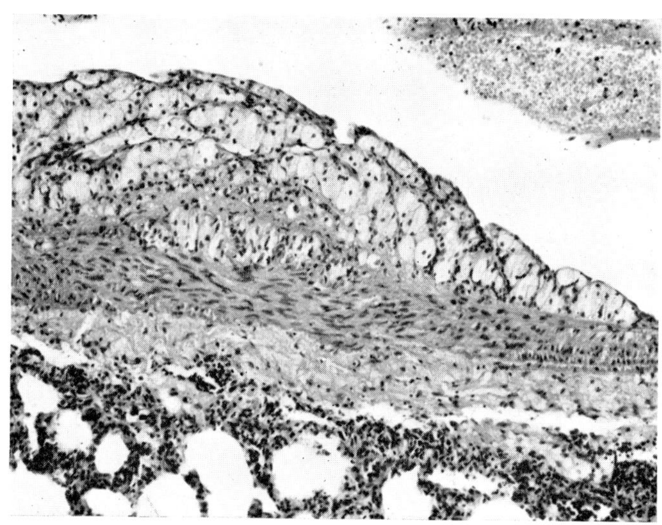

FIG. 35. Section of rabbit's pulmonary artery after 8 weeks of cholesterol feeding. Foam-cells are deposited on the intimal surface in layers alternating with layers of flattened cells resembling endothelium. (I am indebted to Professor I Rannie for this illustration.)

while others lay apparently exposed to the circulating blood. In some instances foam-cells could be seen floating free in the circulating blood especially in the pulmonary arteries, and in some of the pulmonary arteries the deposits of foam-cells were arranged in layers one or two cells thick, alternating with single layers of flattened cells resembling endothelium (fig 35), as if each deposit of cholesterol-bearing cells had been covered with endothelium before the next was laid down.

Most of the lesions consisted mainly of intact foam-cells, but in some of the older ones the foam-cells in the deeper layers had broken down, setting free their contents to form atheromatous masses of cholesterol and lipid debris which closely resembled human atheroma. In some of these, when the lipids were dissolved out, a delicate stroma of ill defined fibres could be seen, which had bound the masses of debris together, but in none of them was there any fibrin deposit or fibrous thickenings of the kind associated with the organisation of mural thrombi.

In one rabbit which had survived the treatment for forty-five weeks there was an enormous accumulation of cholesterol and lipids coating the inner surface of the aorta and forming an extreme thickening with dilatation of the vessel (fig 36). This was something of a freak effect, but it is included in this description because it emphasises in a most striking way how a progressive heaping up of cholesterol deposits on the intimal surface, instead of encroaching

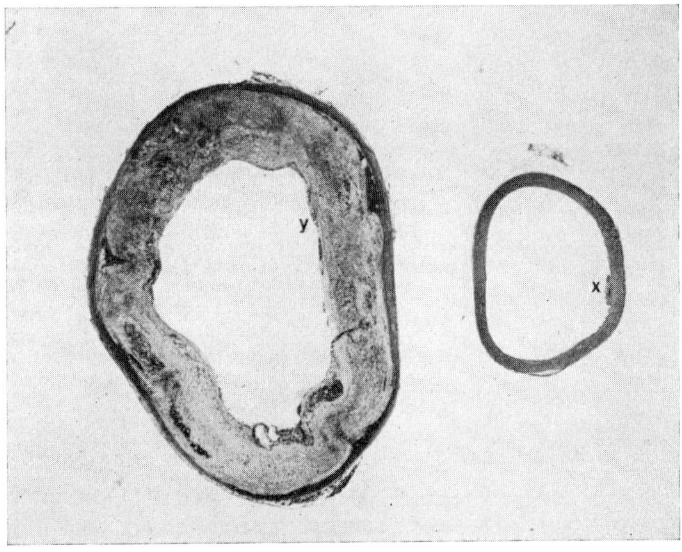

FIG. 36. Aortas from two rabbits which before cholesterol feeding were about the same age and weight, taken from the same region of the thoracic aorta and shown at the same magnification. The artery on the right is from the rabbit killed in the 6th week of treatment and shows a small heap of foam-cells on the intimal surface at x. The artery on the left is from a rabbit which survived the treatment for 45 weeks. Its wall consists almost entirely of cholesterol and fatty debris, the medial coat being represented by the thin dark line on the outer surface. A thin layer of foam-cells are loosely attached to the surface at y. Frozen sections: Sudan III and haemalum, × 10.

on the lumen, causes a progressive stretching of the vessel wall resulting in dilatation of the lumen.

In all the other rabbits the lesions were discrete and nodular and, wherever there was a breakdown of cells, they resembled athero-sclerosis. Up to a point, therefore, the experiments seemed to support the lipid theory in that they showed that raising the level of chol-esterol in the blood resulted in deposits of that substance in the arteries and produced lesions which might be said to be comparable with those of the familial hypercholesterolaemia in man. But the bearing of this on atherosclerosis in general, and on coronary disease in particular, may not be quite so clear and direct as the advocates of the lipid theory would have us believe. In the first place, the rabbits are made to ingest relatively enormous amounts of what is to them a totally unnatural article of diet and, in the second place, much depends on what, exactly, is meant by 'coronary disease' a term which is at present a little vague.

Atherosclerosis and Coronary Disease

According to the lipid theory atherosclerosis is caused by eating too much of certain kinds of fat, and so the treatment of coronary disease involves restricting the dietary intake of fats. This might be justifiable if the term coronary disease simply meant fatty change of the arteries, but it covers more than that. To the clinician it implies narrowing of the arteries and impairment of the coronary circulation leading to what is known as 'coronary heart disease' and we now know that it is not fatty change that causes the narrowing, but thrombosis. As yet there is no clear evidence that thrombosis depends on diet; there may be a connection, it is true, but it seems hardly direct enough to justify restricting ones diet on the strength of it.

To emphasise this very important practical consideration the writer used to exhibit side by side two hearts (fig 37) which were conveniently found one morning in almost consecutive autopsies. One was from a woman of 73 who died from complications of diabetes mellitus, and the other from a man of 31 who, without any known history of cardiovascular disease, dropped dead at his work from coronary occlusion. In the woman's heart there was intense and widespread fatty change in the extramyocardial coronary arteries

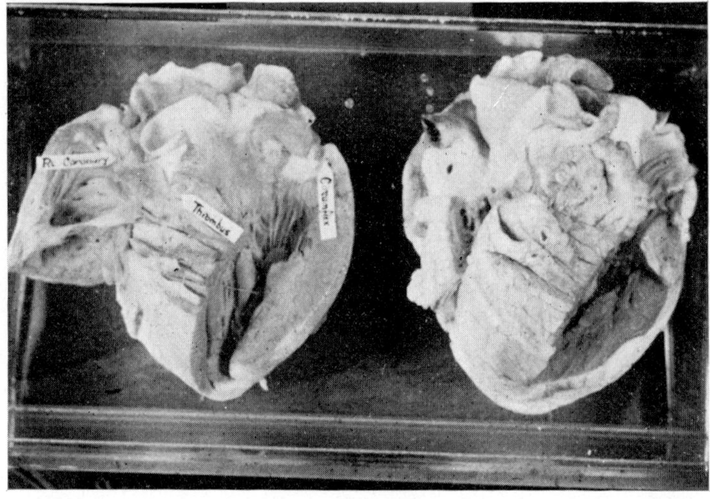

FIG. 37. The heart on the left is from a man of 31 who died suddenly from coronary occlusion, the heart on the right is from a woman of 73 who died from complications of diabetes mellitus.

(fig. 38), probably associated with diabetic lipaemia. In other words, there was severe coronary atherosclerosis, but with it there was a general widening of the arteries of the senile type, so that any circulatory impairment was unlikely. In the man's coronary artery, on the other hand, there was very little fatty change and little sign of disease apart from the one abruptly localised focus of narrowing in the left coronary artery by a dense, fibrous thickening of the kind we have learned to recognise as organised thrombi (fig 39). This was obviously of some standing but there was also a terminal thrombus blocking the lumen at its narrowest part.

Thus, although both hearts might be said to exhibit coronary disease, the respective processes were very different. The woman, had severe coronary atherosclerosis, but it was clinically silent and relatively harmless, whereas the man had fatal coronary occlusion and it was due, not to fatty change but to thrombosis.

Lipids and Thrombosis

It has been suggested that the fatty changes in the arteries promote thrombosis, and one of our first purposes in undertaking the cholesterol experiments was to test this point. The results were

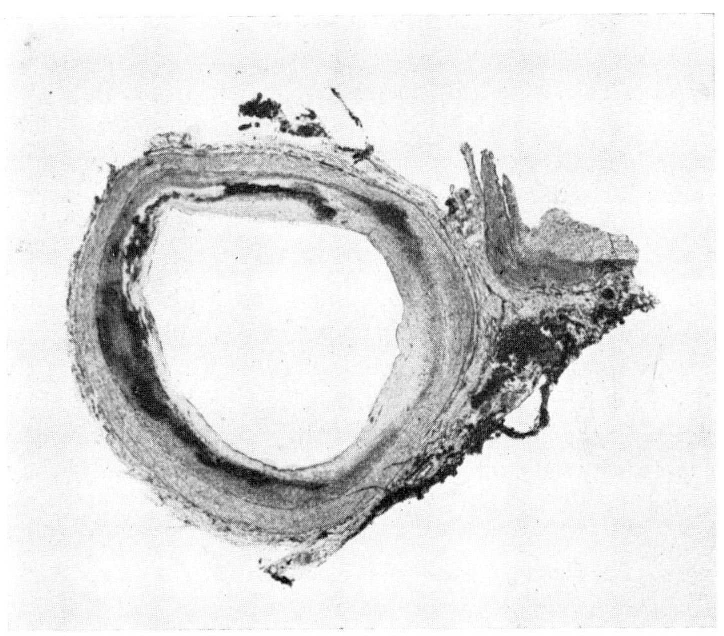

FIG. 38. Left coronary artery from the woman's heart showing senile ectasis. There is diffuse thickening of the intima with much fatty change (black streaking) around the whole circumference of the vessel. In most parts the intima is thicker than the media while the lumen is widened. Frozen section: Sudan III and haemalum, × 15.

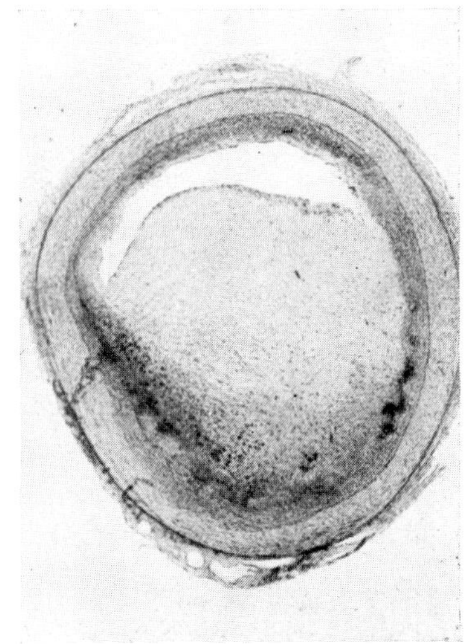

FIG. 39. Left coronary from the man's heart sectioned at the point of occlusion. The lumen is almost totally occluded by a fibrous mass representing an organised thrombus of some standing. From its shape it would appear to have originally occluded the lumen but later retracted. There was a terminal thrombus finally occluding the lumen but this was extremely fragile and was lost in mounting the section. Frozen section: Sudan III and haemalum, × 15.

entirely negative for, in spite of numerous and widespread cholesterol deposits, there was never any fibrin formation in the rabbit's
arteries. This, admittedly, may have been due to the richness in
fibrinolysins of rabbit's blood, but such a complete absence of fibrin
makes it hard to believe that cholesterol has any thrombogenic
effect, just as the complete absence of fibrin deposits in the woman's
arteries makes it hard to believe that the fatty changes in human
arteries promote thrombosis. In fact, the marked absence of a
cellular reaction in most atherosclerotic lesions has been commented
on by more than one observer in the past and it certainly leaves room
for doubts as to the fibrous tissue promoting capacity of the lipids.
To the writer it suggests that the lipids are bland: nevertheless,
where they accumulate in large amounts, they must interfere with
the elasticity and flexibility of the tissues and thus be a contributory
factor in the atherosclerotic process.

There is, of course, the possibility that the lipids exert an
influence through the part they play in the clotting process. Certain
lipids are known to be essential in blood coagulation, and it may
well be that, as Fullerton *et al.* (1953) suggested, alimentary lipaemia
favours fibrin formation. Still (1972) reported the formation of
microthrombi in aortas of hypertensive rats following corticotropin
injections administered in order to raise their endogenous free fatty
acid levels. But it seems to us that, if there is a connection it cannot
be a very straightforward one because mural thrombosis is a focal
lesion, and there must be some local factor in the vessel wall determining when and where the thrombi occur. Clearly the local
factors must be the crucial ones and, as it happens, there is one set
of cholesterol experiments, reported by Harrison in 1933, which
sheds some light on this point.

Cholesterol and Movement

Harrison produced cholesterol lesions in rabbits which had previously been given courses of irradiated ergosterol together with
large amounts of calcium in order to bring about calcification of
their arteries. In some of the animals large segments of their aortic
walls were rigidly immobilised by medial calcification, and when
these animals were subsequently given the cholesterol treatment,
only those parts of the vessel walls that remained free and mobile

developed cholesterol deposits (fig 40), while the immobilised segments escaped. It would surely be hard to find a more striking experimental demonstration of the importance of movement in arterial pathology and it seems surprising that Harrison's observations have received so little attention.

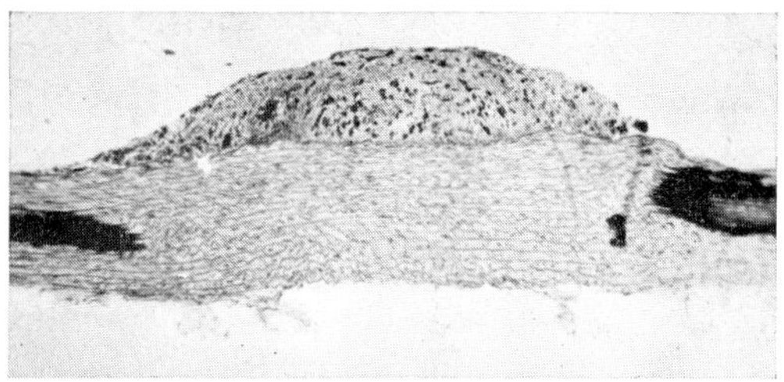

FIG. 40. Section of rabbit aorta showing experimental calcification and a subsequently induced cholesterol lesion. Calcification is represented by dark streaks in media at sides. In these parts the media is thinned and the elastic laminae straightened indicating that the wall was fixed in the stretched position. The cholesterol lesion is confined to the central part where the vessel wall was still free to contract. Frozen section: Sudan III and haemalum, ×40.
(I am indebted to Professor C V Harrison for this illustration.)

On the whole the cholesterol experiments have not taken us very far towards an understanding of atherosclerosis. The sharp differences of opinion that have been expressed on such fundamental questions as the origin of the foam cells in the experimental lesions shows how far we are from solving the problem. Most observers have regarded the foam cells as local endothelial or connective tissue cells which have absorbed cholesterol from the body fluids, but Leary (1949) took them to be liver cells which had been carried to the arteries in the blood stream. Our findings seemed to support Leary in that in some of the cases we saw foam cells apparently being carried in the blood but, whereas Leary thought that they got into the vessel walls by creeping through between the endothelial cells, we had the impression that they were deposited on the intimal surface and then passively incorporated into the intima by a rearrangement of the endothelial lining. It must however, in fairness, be stated that Poole and Florey (1958) have shown sections with foam-cells apparently passing through the endothelium of a rabbit aorta and Still and O'Neal (1962) obesrved the same in a rat aorta. Thus, instead of explaining atheroma, the cholesterol experiments have only presented us with another problem and one which may, or may not, have a bearing on the human disease.

Mitchell and Schwartz, in their excellent monograph (Arterial Diseases, 1965), expressed the opinion that the cholesterol experiments have confused rather than clarified the various issues and, one might add, retarded the progress of the enquiry. By encouraging investigators to choose the experimental approach rather than the more prosaic study of the human lesions they have set a fashion which has resulted in the amassing of a large amount of information about fats and very little about arteries, even the fact of pulsation having been largely forgotten. There may be no end to the planning of studies to show that this or that article of diet may raise the lipid content of the blood and increase the amount of fats in the arteries, but such studies are of doubtful value so long as it has yet to be shown exactly what harm the fats do in the arteries. What is now needed is a return to the study of the human lesion.

Chapter Ten

Effects of Ageing

In the aorta and its main branches there is an irregular but progressive thickening of the intima from birth to old age and, since it is universal in man, it is regarded as natural. Nevertheless, in those who live to old age, it commonly gives rise to stiffenings which cause the discord and disruptions characteristic of atherosclerosis, in which case it must be classified as pathological. Jorés (1902) believed that the intimal thickenings of atheroma were simply continuations of the normal growth and we are consequently confronted with the question: what then is the histogenesis of the normal growth?

Development of the Intima

In early fetal life the aortic intima consists of little more than a layer of endothelium lying directly on the internal elastic lamina, but at birth a subendothelial layer of fibrous tisse has already formed and begun to increase. By adult life the intima has become a compound layer with a musculo-elastic zone externally and a fibro-elastic zone internally, and it is this internal, subendothelial zone, sometimes called the hyperplastic layer of Jorés, that increases with age. In the peripheral arteries the intima is a simpler structure, usually consisting of a subendothelial, fibrous layer only, which also increases with age, especially in the more proximal arteries.

Whilst the normal development of the intima is generally assumed to be by a proliferation of connective tissue cells, pathological thickenings, in some instances at least, are acknowledged to be products of thrombosis, and it might therefore be expected that in the adult aorta signs of this duality would sometimes be apparent, but they never are. We have seen how in atherosclerosis the inner layers of the intima are sometimes composed of organising thrombi, but when the organisation is completed nothing remains to reveal their original nature and they merge imperceptibly into the original intimal tissues as if they were the same. It is conceivable, therefore, that the normal intima, or at least the intima that increases with age, may also be a product of thrombosis.

Reaction to Injury

In 1952 McLetchie wrote: 'With the increasing imperfections of age an increasing deposit from the circulating blood is to be expected and hence an increasing build-up of intimal thickenings by a slow assimilation and organisation of the deposits'. This sounded fanciful at the time, but our findings ever since have borne it out. There is little doubt that minute injuries occur in the arterial lining from time to time. Poole, Sanders and Florey (1958) drew attention to the occurence of mitoses in the aortic endothelium as evidence of such injuries, and Wright (1968) reported the frequency of mitoses in the endothelium around the openings of the intercostal branches of the normal guinea-pig aorta. It seems justifiable therefore to assume that, even in normal life, small injuries occur, and one naturally thinks of microthrombi as part of the repair process. This is discussed in a valuable communication by French (1971). We have only recently come to realise how common microthrombi are. Most of them are extremely thin and inconspicuous, probably consisting almost entirely of platelets, and the more we see of them the stronger becomes the impression that they are the substance of which the intimal thickenings of ageing are composed.

So long as intimal thickenings are fairly even and uniform they cause little discord, and may be hardly noticeable, but they never are quite uniform. Even in fetal life, as Robertson (1960) has shown, the intima around the openings of the intercostal arteries in the aorta tends to be thicker than elsewhere, and this must constitute a potential source of discord. It seems significant, therefore, that these are the points where Wright noted an outstanding frequency of mitotic figures in the rat's aorta. They are also the parts where, as pointed out on page 9, pulse movements are theoretically likely to be accentuated and where, in the human aorta, the earliest atherosclerotic lesions commonly appear.

It has been suggested that injuries to the arterial lining may be caused by eddies or turbulences in the blood stream and, whilst this cannot be discounted, it must be realised that, as compared with the movements imposed on the vessel walls by the pulse pressure, turbulences in the blood stream must be mild. It has, of course, always to be borne in mind that, whilst we think of pulse movements as the disrupting agents, it is actually the thickenings of the intima interfering with the pulse movements that cause the disruptions.

Hazards of Ageing

For as long as autopsies have been practiced it has been recognised that in those who live beyond middle-age atherosclerosis is practically inevitable. Accordingly the disease used to be regarded as trivial, but later, owing to its association with coronary disease, it came to be looked on as 'the great killer'. This, however, is not quite justifiable because, as explained in the foregoing chapter, it is not atherosclerosis that causes coronary occlusion, but the gross thrombosis which sometimes complicates atherosclerosis. The atherosclerotic lesion is itself relatively harmless or, at worst, its ill effects are usually deferred until late in life. In old age complications may arise, some of them with disastrous results, an example being dissecting aneurysm. Among the thirty-five consecutive autopsies investigated for haemosiderin (p 45), there were two on individuals of over 70 in whom blood from atheromatous foci in the intima had tracked out to the medial coats where they formed haematomas (fig 41). In one of them, as will be seen in the

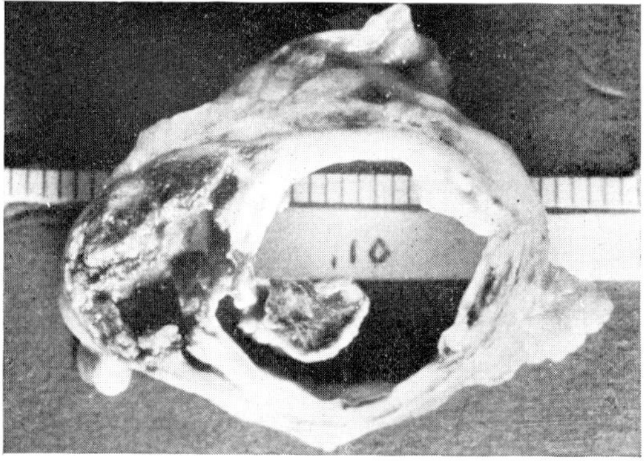

FIG. 41. Cross section of abdominal aorta from a man of 85 showing a haematoma extending from the intima into the media. There is also a rupture of the intimal surface making a direct passage from the lumen to the medial haematoma. There is also a polypoid thrombus in the lumen arising at the point of rupture.

illustration, there was also ulceration of the intima, making a free passage from the lumen into the media, but in neither of them was there any tracking of blood along the layers of the media. The lesions had not actually developed to the stage of dissecting aneurysm formation, but the specimens provided striking demonstrations of how such aneurysms may arise, and the occurrence of two such cases in so small a sequence of autopsies makes it surprising that dissecting aneurysms are not more common in old age.

A more common ill-effect of advanced atherosclerosis is high systolic blood pressure. Often in old age the aorta is so beset with atherosclerotic plaques that its elasticity is largely destroyed and its buffering effect which normally shields the peripheral arteries from the sharp rises of pressure in systole is lost. There is then the danger of rupture of the smaller arteries and haemorrhage, especially in the cerebral system.

Chapter Eleven

Prevention of Atherosclerosis

In planning the prevention of a disease one must have clearly in mind the nature of the process and exactly what is to be prevented. For the last thirty years our chief aim in connection with atherosclerosis has been the prevention of fatty infiltration of the arteries by restricting the dietary intake of fats on the assumption that they are the damaging agents, but we now know that the problem is not so simple as this. Underlying the fatty changes in atherosclerosis there is a much more destructive process involving splitting and tearing apart of the layers of the intima with recurring haemorrhages, and these have the unmistakable marks of a mechanical process. If we consider the dynamic forces to which the walls of the aorta and its branches are exposed, and the movements they are forced to undergo, we cannot escape the conclusion that the changes are connected with pulsation. The early writers ascribed them to excessive pulsation but we now know that excessive movements are not necessary. When the intima of a pulsating artery becomes thickened by fibrous tissue it loses its flexibility and can no longer conform in the usual way even to the normal pulse movements. Consequently, disruption of the kind we see in atherosclerosis is bound to follow.

Prevention of Thrombosis

There is reason to believe that most fibrous thickenings of the intima in atherosclerosis are products of mural thrombi, and it is therefore to the prevention of thrombosis rather than fatty change we should turn our attention, but here we are faced with a dilemma. We have learned to dread coronary thrombosis, 'the great killer' as it has been called, but at the same time we know that thrombosis also plays an essential part in the repair of injuries to the arterial lining and is a part of the haemostatic mechanism with which we may not lightly interfere. We must now recognise two categories of arterial thrombi, both consisting of fibrin and platelets but in differing proportions, and of very different significance. There are the microthrombi which consist mostly of platelets and are often so small as to be overlooked, and there are the fibrin thrombi which form the large masses we associate with coronary occlusion. The two constitute, as it were, the arterial counterparts of the simple vegetative endocarditis on the one hand, and the malignant or infective endocarditis on the other, and their respective causes may be similar, but there is no doubt as to which of the two we should aim to prevent. Obviously it is the excessive fibrin that is the dangerous element.

Much information has been acquired regarding thrombosis in the last ten years. It has been reviewed by Nicolaides (1975) and by the many writers who have contributed to 'Clinics in Haematology', including especially the volume on Platelet Diseases, edited by O'Brien (1973) and that on Blood Coagulation and Fibrinolysis, edited by Douglas (1973). Yet we are still uncertain as to which of the many factors involved in thrombosis is responsible for excessive fibrin formation; whether it depends on a hypercoagulability of the blood, or on a failure of some anti-coagulant factor, or on a depressed fibrinolytic potential of the blood is still to be determined.

Fibrinolysis

In 1948 Mole suggested that atherosclerosis might be due to a deficiency in fibrinolysis. He noted the continuous production of fibrinogen in the liver and concluded that there must be a constant laying down of fibrin somewhere in the body and a constant removal of it by fibrinolysis. Such a process, if we could exploit it, might be the ideal therapeutic agent against the dangers of excessive fibrin because, whilst it does not interfere with the natural fibrin formation, it can remove unwanted fibrin before this becomes a danger.

Astrup, who has studied fibrinolysis intensively (1947, 1956 and 1968) has postulated a haemostatic balance between thromboplastic and fibrinolytic agents governing the healing process. He visualized the constant occurrence of minute injuries to the arterial lining and their repair involving deposits of fibrin which in due course have to be removed to restore normal structures. He has demonstrated the production of a lytic agent (plasmin) by the activation of an enzyme (plasminogen) in certain tissues, and Todd (1959) has confirmed this histologically. Using his modification of Astrup's fibrin plate method, Todd demonstrated the presence of an activator in some of the endothelial cells of veins and pulmonary arteries, and it seems possible that these, and other cells like them, may be the agents which determine whether mural thrombi are to be resolved or converted into fibrous thickenings of the intima.

It has been observed that the fibrinolytic potential of the blood is not entirely outside our control. It is increased by exercise (Douglas, 1962) and tends to rise after surgical operations (Macfarlane, 1937). It tends, on the other hand, to be reduced after fatty meals (Fullerton, 1953), again suggesting a relationship of atherosclerosis to the lipid metabolism. It has also been suggested that fibrinolysis is linked with racial factors, Shaper (1972) having drawn attention to the higher fibrinolytic potential in the bloods of natives of New Guinea than those of white Australians, as reported by Grace, Sennett and Whyte (1970), and suggested that this might account for the lower incidence of atherosclerosis in New Guinea.

Physical Activity

There are indications that the dangers of atherosclerosis may be reduced by physical activity. Morris and his co-workers (1956) found that coronary disease of middle life was commoner in sedentary workers than in those whose occupations demanded greater physical activity and that sudden death from coronary disease was commoner in London bus drivers than in conductors whose occupation was more strenuous. These findings emphasise what we have known all along, namely that exercise is good for one, but whether it does good by increasing the fibrinolytic potential of the blood or by preserving the elasticity and flexibility of the arteries or by some other means we do not know. During exercise, pulse pressure is increased and pulse movements accentuated, so that one might reasonably expect mechanical damage to be increased, but this does not always follow. Presumably it is only in arteries that have lost their normal flexibility that pulse movements bring about disruption, in which case the best regime would be adequate exercise for the young, to maintain the flexibility of their arteries, and more restricted exercise for older subjects whose arteries are stiffer and therefore susceptible to mechanical damage.

Hypertension

It is difficult to know to what extent pulse movements may be affected by hypertension but Mills, Moffatt and Paterson (1958) and

6

Paterson, Mills and Lockwood (1960) have emphasised that atherosclerosis with intimal haemorrhage is especially prominent in the aortas of subjects who have been hypertensive. This coincides with our own impression and it would suggest that the mechanical factor responsible for the disruption in atherosclerosis is increased in hypertension. It also seems likely that tension itself may be a dangerous factor especially in advanced atherosclerosis. It was suggested on page 37 that coronary occlusion may be relieved by detachment and shrinkage of the occluding thrombus, provided always that the vessel wall is relaxed enough to allow blood to pass. Presumably a high vascular tension would counteract relaxation and so reduce the chances of survival in cases of coronary occlusion. From the pathologist's point of view these are merely conjectures but they are largely borne out by the clinical evidence which seems to indicate that the reduction of hypertension should be a first consideration in the protection against the dangers of atherosclerosis.

The Future Prospect

More information is needed before we can finally elucidate the problem of atherosclerosis and our progress in that direction will depend on our choosing the right lines for investigation. One of the purposes of this monograph has been to show that the lipid theory has not been the best of guides in that direction. No doubt lipids play a part in the process; loading the vessel walls with fat is bound to reduce their resilience, but preoccupation with the fats has blinded observers to other, more important features of the process. The splitting and tearing apart of the layers of the intima and the haemorrhages into the tears have been largely obscured by the fats and consequently the essential nature of the process has been overlooked.

The new evidence presented in the foregoing chapters has shed a fresh light on the problem, pointing in the first place to the need for more information about the functional activity of arteries. It has also enabled us to see something of the limitations in the prospect of prevention. The thickening of the intima which goes with ageing obviously involves stiffening which must sooner or later lead to disruption so that in those who live to middle age atherosclerosis is unavoidable. Fortunately it is a mild condition with which one can live comfortably; nevertheless it is a dangerous one since it is commonly associated with gross thrombosis involving narrowing or occlusion of the arteries. There is reason to hope that we may in time learn to control fibrin formation and so perhaps reduce the dangers, but that is about the most we can hope to do. To think of preventing atherosclerosis itself is to shut ones eyes to the nature of the condition. It is a product of ageing and, as Aschoff (1938) remarked, there is no remedy for old age.

Chapter Twelve

Summary and Conclusions

It may be of assistance if the writer summarises his interpretation of the atherosclerotic process in a series of simple drawings, showing also the effects of postmortem contraction on the histological appearances. Each drawing illustrates a stage in the development of a hard fibrous plaque (left) and a soft atheromatous nodule (right).

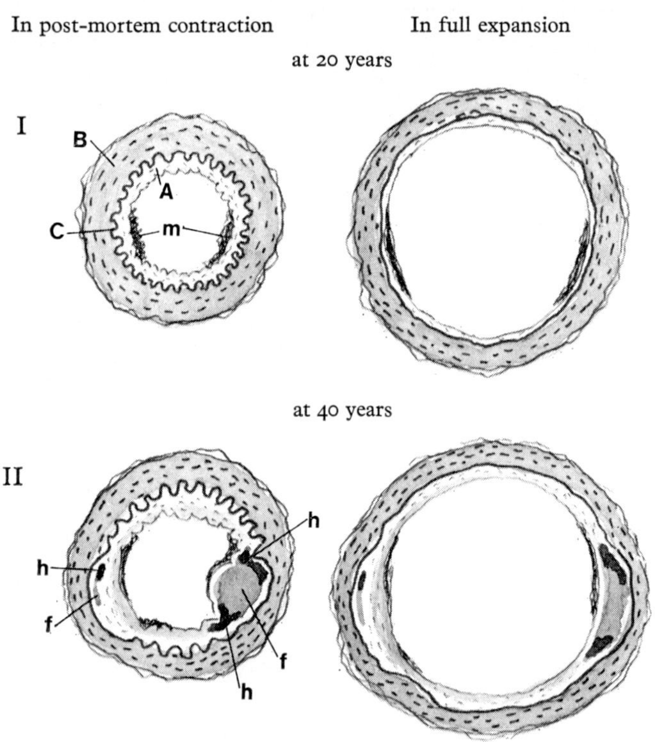

A intima   B media   C internal elastic lamina   f fatty deposit
h haemorrhage   m microthrombus   t gross thrombus   u ulceration

Microthrombi occur at as early as three years of age and continue to occur throughout life (I). By forty years their repeated incorporation into the intima results in irregular fibrous thickenings which are too stiff to comply in the normal way with pulse movements and so cause disruption and haemorrhage (II). The extravasated blood disintegrates leaving fatty deposits which accumulate progressively, and when haemorrhages are frequent and profuse the deposits predominate whilst the fibrous tissue is relatively sparse, with the result that the thickenings are soft and friable. In such

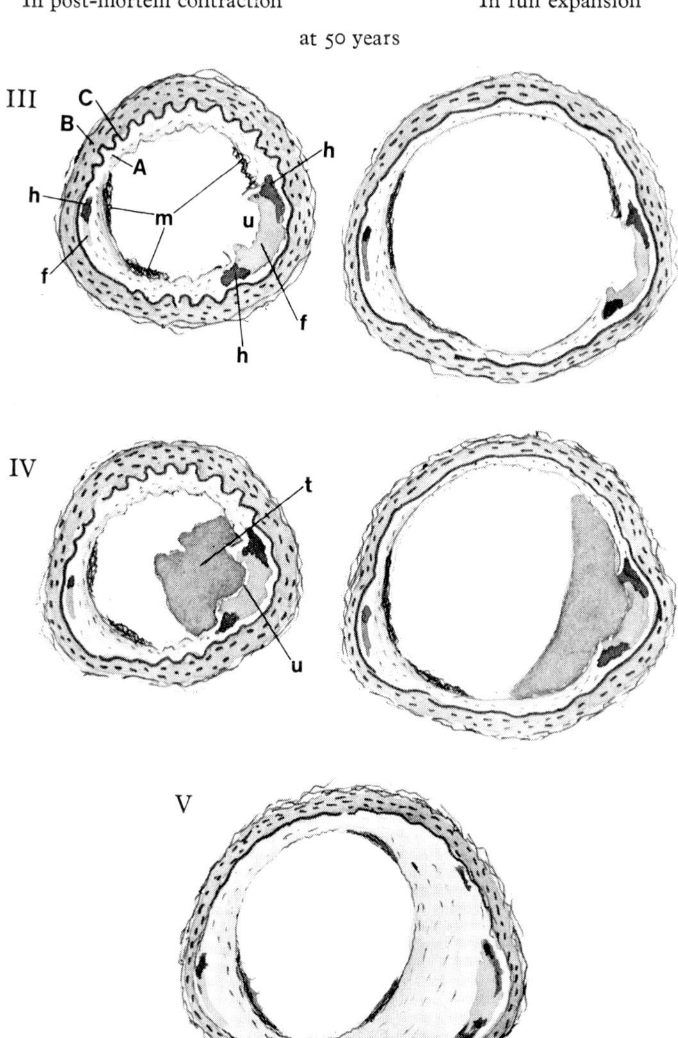

circumstance the surface layers are liable to be torn away leaving ulcers (III) which promote gross mural thrombosis (IV). The thrombi become organised and form fibrous thickenings which narrow the arteries (V) and destroy their elasticity.

The foregoing interpretation of atherosclerosis presents the fats in a fresh light. For the last quarter of a century they have been regarded as the cause of the disease whereas they are now represented as playing a subsidiary role. The basis of this change of view is the recognition of pulse movements. We know that the walls of the aorta and its larger branches are elastic and are stretched and recoil with each heart beat. With this in mind it is easy to see how in these vessels the incorporation into the intima of layers of relatively stiff fibrous tissue, such as are formed by the organisation of mural thrombi, must lead to disruption and haemorrhage. It would appear that all the essential changes in atherosclerosis can be accounted for in this way.

References

ANITSCHKOW, N. & CHALATOW, S. (1913). Über experimentelle Cholesterinsteatose und ihre Bedeutung fur die Entstehung einiger pathologischer Prozesse. *Centrelbl. f. allg. Path.* **24,** 1.

ASCHOFF, L. (1924). *Lectures on Pathology.* New York. Paul B. Hoeber.

ASCHOFF, L. (1938). Zur normalen und pathologischen Anatomie des Greisenalters. *Med. Klin.* **33** & **34** (January–June).

ASTRUP, T. (1956). The biological significance of fibrinolysis. *Lancet,* **ii,** 565.

ASTRUP, T. (1968). Blood coagulation, fibrinolysis and the development of the thrombogenic theory of atherosclerosis. *Le Role de la Paroi Arterielle dans l'Athérogénèse,* **2,** 535. Paris.

ASTRUP, T. (1947). Fibrinolysis in the animal organism. *Nature,* **159,** 681.

BARKHAN, P., SILVER, M. J. & O'KEEFE, L. M. (1961). *Blood Platelets.* Boston: Little, Brown & Co. Quoted by Mitchell and Schwartz, 1965.

BOYD, A. M. (1938). Thromoangeitis obliterans. *St Barts. Hosp. Rep.* **71,** 151.

BURTON, A. C. (1967). Haemodynamics as related to structure. *Cowdry's Arteriosclerosis,* 2nd edition, p. 66. Springfield, Ill.: Charles C. Thomas.

CLARK, E., GRAEF, I. & CHASIS, H. (1936). Thrombosis of the aorta and coronary arteries with special reference to 'fibrinoid' lesions. *Arch. Path.* **22,** 183.

COOK, T. A., SALMO, N. A. M. & YATES, P. O. (1975). The elasticity of the internal lamina. *J. Path.* **117,** 253.

CRAWFORD, T. & LEVENE, C. (1952). The incorporation of fibrin in the aortic intima. *J. Path. Bact.* **64,** 523.

CRAWFORD, T. & WOOLF, N. (1968). Changes occurring in experimentally produced aortic mural thrombi. *Le Role de la Paroi Arterielle dans l'Athérogénèse,* vol. 2. Paris.

DAVIES, M. J., BALLANTINE, SANDRA J., ROBERTSON, W. B. & WOOLF, N. (1975). The ultrastructure of experimental mural thrombi in the pig aorta. *J. Path.* **117,** 75.

DIBLE, J. H. (1966). *The Pathology of Limb Ischaemia.* Edinburgh: Oliver & Boyd.

DOUGLAS, A. S. (1962). *Anticoagulant Therapy.* Oxford: Blackwell.

DOUGLAS, A. S. (1973). *Clinics in Haematology: Blood Coagulation and Fibrinolysis.* London: W. B. Saunders & Co.

DUGUID, J. B. (1926). Atheroma of the aorta. *J. Path. Bact.* **29,** 371.

DUGUID, J. B. (1946). Thrombosis as a factor in the pathogenesis of coronary atherosclerosis. *J. Path. Bact.* **58,** 207.

DUGUID, J. B. (1948). Thrombosis as a factor in the pathogenesis of aortic atherosclerosis. *J. Path. Bact.* **60,** 57.

DUGUID, J. B. (1952). The arterial lining. *Lancet,* **ii,** 207.

DUGUID, J. B. & ROBERTSON, W. B. (1957). Mechanical factors in atherosclerosis. *Lancet,* **i,** 1205.

FRENCH, J. E. (1968). Blood platelets and the arterial wall. *Le Role de la Paroi Arterielle dans l'Athérogénèse.* Paris.

FRENCH, J. E. (1971). Atherogenesis and thrombosis. *Semin. Haematol.*, vol. 8, no. 1 (January).

FULLERTON, H. W., DAVIE, W. J. A. & ANASTASOPOULAS, G. (1953). Relationship of alimentary lipaemia to blood coagulability. *Brit. Med. J.* **ii,** 250.

GEIRINGER, E. (1951). Intimal vascularisation and atherosclerosis. *J. Path. Bact.* **63,** 201.

GHANI, A. R. (1969). The role of blood mononuclear cells in the organisation of mural thrombi. *J. Path. Bact.* **97,** 11.

GHANI, A. R. & TIBBS, J. D. (1962). Role of blood-borne cells in organisation of mural thrombi. *Brit. Med. J.* **i,** 1244.

GITLIN, D. & CRAIG, J. M. (1957). Variation in staining characteristics of human fibrin. *Amer. J. Path.* **33,** 267.

GRACE, C. S., SINNETT, P. & WHYTE, H. M. (1970). Blood fibrinolysis and coagulation in New Guineans and Australians. *Australasian Annls. of Med.* **19,** 329.

HAND, R. A. & CHANDLER, A. B. (1962). Arteriosclerotic metamorphosis of autologous pulmonary thrombo-emboli in the rabbit. *Amer. J. Path.* **40,** 469.

HARRISON, C. V. (1933). Experimental arterial disease produced by cholesterol and vitamin D. *J. Path. Bact.* **36,** 447.

HARRISON, C. V. (1948). Experimental pulmonary arteriosclerosis. *J. Path. Bact.* **60,** 289.

HEARD, B. E. (1949). Mural thrombosis in the renal artery and its relation to atherosclerosis. *J. Path. Bact.* **61,** 635.

HEARD, B. E. (1952). An experimental study of thickening of the pulmonary arteries of rabbits produced by organisation of fibrin. *J. Path. Bact.* **64,** 13.

HOLMAN, R. L., McGILL, H. C., STRONG, J. P. & GEER, J. C. (1958). The natural history of atherosclerosis. *Amer. J. Path.* **34,** 209.

HORN, H. & FINKELSTEIN, L. E. (1940). Arteriosclerosis of the coronary arteries and the mechanism of their occlusion. *Amer. Heart J.* **19,** 655.

IGNATOWSKI, A. (1909). Über die Wirkung des tierschen Eiweisses auf die Aorta und die parenchymatosen Organe der Kaninchen. *Virchows Arch.* **198,** 248.

JORES, L. (1903). *Wesen und Entwicklung der Arteriosclerose.* Wiesbaden: J. F. Bergmann.

JØRGENSEN, L., ROWSEL, H. C., TORSTEIN, H. & MUSTARD, J. F. (1967). Resolution and organisation of platelet-rich mural thrombi in carotid arteries of swine. *Amer. J. Path.* **51,** 681.

LEARY, T. (1949). Crystalline ester cholesterol and atherosclerosis. *Arch. Path.* **47,** 1.

LENDRUM, A. C., FRASER, D. S., SLIDDERS, W. & HENDERSON, R. (1962). Studies on the character and standing of fibrin. *J. Clin. Path.* **15,** 401.

LEVENE, C. I. (1955). Electron-microscopy of atheroma. *Lancet,* **ii,** 1216.

LEVENE, C. I. (1956). (a) The early lesions of atheroma in the coronary arteries. (b) The pathogenesis of atheroma of the coronary arteries. *J. Path. Bact.* **72,** 79 and 83.

LIKAR, I. N., LIKAR, LYDIA, ROBINSON, R. W. & GOUVELIS, A. (1969). Microthrombi and intimal thickening in bovine coronary arteries. *Arch. Path.* **87,** 148.

LISTER, J. (1879). Influence of position upon local circulation. *Brit. Med. J.* **i,** 923.

McDONALD, D. A. (1960). *Blood Flow in Arteries.* London: Arnold.

MACFARLANE, R. G. (1937). Fibrinolysis following operations. *Lancet,* **i,** 10.

McLETCHIE, N. G. B. (1952). The pathogenesis of atheroma. *Amer. J. Path.* **28,** 413.

MACWILLIAM, J. A. (1902). On the properties of arterial and venous walls. *Proc. Roy. Soc.* **70,** 109.

MACWILLIAM, J. A. & MACKIE, A. H. (1908). Arteries, normal and pathological. *Brit. Med. J.* **ii,** 1477.

MALLORY, F. B. (1912–13). *The Infectious Lesions of Blood Vessels.* Harvey Lectures. Philadelphia: Lippencot & Co.

MILLS, JEAN., MOFFATT, T. & PATERSON, J. C. (1958). Incidence of intimal haemorrhage of the aorta in normotensive and hypertensive men. *Lab. Invest.* **7,** 608.

MITCHELL, J. R. A. & SCHWARTZ, C. J. (1965). *Arterial Disease.* Oxford: Blackwell.

MOLE, R. H. (1948). Fibrinolysin and the fluidity of the blood post mortem. *J. Path. Bact.* **60,** 413.

MONTGOMERY, G. L. (1957–58). Problems in the pathology of coronary artery disease. *Lectures on the Scientific Basis of Medicine,* vol 7.

MORGAN, A. D. (1956). *The Pathogenesis of Coronary Occlusion.* Oxford: Blackwell.

MORRIS, J. N., HEADY, J. A. & RAFFLE, P. A. B. (1956). Physique of London busmen. *Lancet,* **ii,** 569.

MUSTARD, J. F., PACKHAM, MARIAN A., NISHIZAWA, E. E. & ROWSELL, H. C. (1968). The relationship between thrombosis and atherosclerosis. *Le Role de la Paroi Arterielle dans l'Athérogénèse.* Paris.

NICOLAIDES, A. N. (1975). *Thromboembolism.* Lancaster: Med. and Tech. Publishing Co.

O'BRIEN, J. R. (1973). *Clinics in Haematology: Platelet Disorders.* London: W. B. Saunders & Co.

O'BRIEN, J. R. (1968). Effects of salicylates on human platelets. *Lancet,* **i,** 779.

PATERSON, J. C. (1936). Vascularisation and haemorrhage of the intima of arteriosclerotic coronary arteries. *Arch. Path.* **22,** 313.

PATERSON, J. C., MILLS, JEAN & MOFFATT, T. (1957). Vascularisation of early atherosclerotic plaques. *Arch. Path.* **64,** 129.

PATERSON, J. C., MILLS, JEAN & LOCKWOOD, C. H. (1960). The role of hypertension in the progression of atherosclerosis. *Canada M. A. J.* **82,** 65.

PATERSON, J. C., MOFFATT, T. & MILLS, JEAN (1956). Haemosiderin deposition in early atherosclerotic plaques. *Arch. Path.* **61,** 496.

PICKERING, G. (1963). Arteriosclerosis and atherosclerosis. *Amer. J. Med.* **34,** 7.

POOLE, J. C. F., SANDERS, A. G. & FLOREY, H. W. (1958). Regeneration of aortic endothelium. *J. Path. Bact.* **75,** 133.

POOLE, J. C. F. & FLOREY, H. W. (1958). Changes in the endothelium of the aorta and behaviour of macrophages in experimental atheroma of rabbits. *J. Path. Bact.* **75,** 245.

RANNIE, I. (1956). Experimental cholesterol atherosclerosis. *Proc. Nutr. Soc.* **15,** 61.

RANNIE, I. (1946). Thrombosis in relation to atherosclerosis. *Biological Aspects of Occlusive Vascular Disease.* Ed. Chalmers and Gresham, p. 322.

RANNIE, I. & DUGUID, J. B. (1953). Pathogenesis of cholesterol arteriosclerosis in the rabbit. *J. Path. Bact.* **66,** 395.

ROBERTSON, J. N. (1960). Stress zones in fetal arteries. *J. Clin. Path.* **13,** 133.

ROKITANSKY, C. (1852). *A Manual of Pathological Anatomy,* vol. iv, p. 261. Translated by George M. Day for the Sydenham Society.

SCHWARTZ, C. J. & MITCHELL, J. R. A. (1962). The morphology, terminology and pathogenesis of arterial plaques. *Postgrad. Med. J.* **38,** 25.

SHAPER, A. G. (1972). Cardiovascular disease in the tropics—IV coronary heart disease. *Brit. Med. J.* **ii,** 32.

STILL, W. J. S. and O'NEAL, R. M. (1962). Electron microscopic study of experimental atherosclerosis in the rat. *Amer. J. Path.* **40,** 21.

STILL, W. J. S. (1972). Arterial thrombosis induced by hypertension and fatty acid mobilisation. *Arch. Path.* **94,** 23.

STILL, W. J. S. (1970). Hyperlipaemia and the arterial intima of the hypertensive rat. *Arch. Path.* **89,** 392.

STILL, W. J. S. (1968). The pathogenesis of intimal thickenings produced by hypertension in large arteries in the rat. *Lab. Invest.* **19,** 84.

STILL, W. J. S. & BOULT, E. H. (1957). Electron-microscopic appearance of fibrin in thin sections. *Nature,* **179,** 868.

STILL, W. J. S., GHANI, A. R. & DENNISON, SUSAN (1967). The organisation of isolated mural thrombi in aortic grafts. *Amer. J. Path.* **51,** 1013.

THOMA, R. (1886). Uber die Abhangigkeit der Bindegewebsneubildung in der Arterienintima von der mechanischen Bedingungen des Blutumlaufs. *Virchows Arch.* **104,** 209.

TODD, A. S. (1959). The histological localisation of fibrinolysin activator. *J. Path. Bact.* **78,** 281.

TODD, A. S. (1960). The tissue activator of plasminogen and thrombosis. *Thrombosis and Anticoagulent Therapy.* W. Walker, Edinburgh: Livingstone.

VIRCHOW, R. (1856). *Phlogose und Thrombose im Gefass-system. Gesammelte Abhanglungen zur wissenschaftlichen Medicin.* Frankfurt: Meidingerson. and Co.

WIGGERS, J. C. (1928). *The Pressure Pulses in the Cardiovascular System.* London: Longmans Green.

WILLIAMS, G. (1955). Experimental arterial thrombosis. *J. Path. Bact.* **69,** 199.

WINTERNITZ, M. C., THOMAS, R. M. & LECOMPTE, P. M. (1938). *The Biology of Arteriosclerosis.* Springfield: Thomas.

WOOLF, N. & CRAWFORD, T. (1960). Fatty streaking in the aortic intima studied by an immuno-histological technique. *J. Path. Bact.* **80,** 405.

WRIGHT, H. P. (1968). Endothelial mitoses around aortic branches in normal guinea-pigs. *Nature,* **220,** 78.

ZIEGLER, E. (1896–97). *Special Pathological Anatomy*. Translated and edited by MacAlister and Cattell. London: Macmillan & Co.

ZINSERLING, W. D. (1925). Untersuchungen uber atherosklerose. *Virchows Arch.* **255,** 677.

ZUCKER, MARJORIE B. & PETERSON, JANE (1970). Effect of acetylsalicylic acid and other nonsteroidal anti-inflammatory agents on human blood platelets. *J. Labor and Clin. Med.* **76,** 66.

Acknowledgements

I owe an incalculable debt of gratitude to the many teachers and colleagues who have helped me in this work over the last half century, to Professor T Shennan who launched me on it in the first place and to Professor E H Kettle whose example was such an inspiration in my early days in pathology and to Drs Maisie Duggan, J Gough, C V Harrison, F Magarey, Jo Boissard, E Lichtenberger, W B Robertson, G S Anderson, C Levene, A S Todd, W J S Still, F Storring, I Rannie and others who have helped me to maintain what I hope was a balanced view of the problem of arterial pathology. I am especially indebted to Professor Egon Lichtenberger, Professor C V Harrison and Professor I Rannie for the loan of illustrations and to Professors A R Currie, A L Stalker and G Smith for the hospitality of their laboratories in recent months and to Professor A S Douglas for his help with the more recent works on blood coagulation and fibrinolysis. But my greatest debt is to the many laboratory technicians who have carried out so much of the essential part of this research, work which I was incapable of doing myself. Most closely associated with me were Mr J Napper in Cardiff and Mr A E Young in Newcastle, both of whom were my friends. Their technical knowledge and skill were a constant marvel to me, and I doubt if this work would ever have reached its present state without them. Finally, I am greatly indebted to my old friend Professor J M Peterson for his frequent help and advice in physiological matters and for his help with the construction of this monograph. This publication has been made possible by a generous grant from the Wellcome Trust to whom I offer my grateful thanks.

JBD

Index